PRESSED

INTO CARE

Words to uplift adult children of aging parents

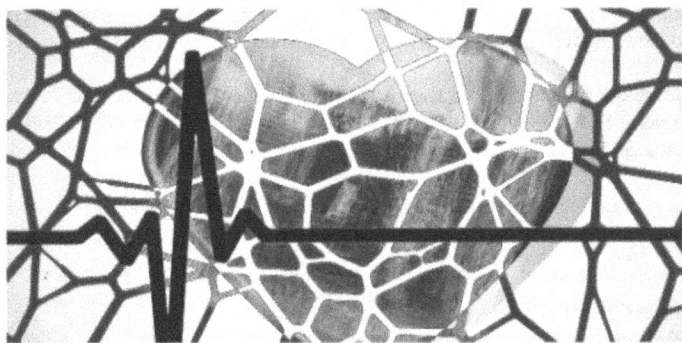

Julie-Allyson Ieron

For Mom,

Who set the caregiving bar high for me.

Please don't follow through

on your threat to write a devotional

for parents caring for their aging children.

I love you always!

Julie

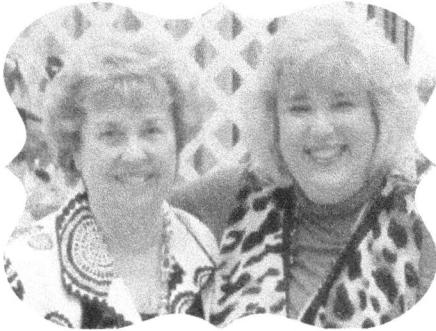

Contents

Welcome from the Author...7

Day 1: Treasured by God..11

Day 2: Precious, Short-lived Solitude...........................15

Day 3: Who's With Me?...17

Day 4: Our Only Source of Strength............................21

Day 5: A Gethsemane Request....................................25

Day 6: Christ's Passion for Our Saddest Times.................29

Day 7: He Is Risen!..33

Day 8: No Better Helper...37

Day 9: So Very Close..41

Day 10: Overwhelmed!...45

Day 11: Cling to This...49

Day 12: Hide and Seek...53

Day 13: When the Well Is Dry......................................57

Day 14: Here We Go Again!..59

Day 15: Answered Prayer...63

Day 16: A Degree I Don't Want...................................67

Day 17: Help!..73

Day 18: Entrusted...77

Day 19: Snow Day...81

Day 20: Word from My Compassionate Lord......................85

Day 21: Jesus, the Caregiver..............................87

Day 22: The Waiting Game.................................91

Day 23: Mom, My Best Friend.............................95

Day 24: Power and Weakness.............................99

Day 25: Hefty Price to Pay................................101

Day 26: Relentless Pursuit of God.....................107

Day 27: The Wind Ceased.................................111

Day 28: Email from God.....................................115

Day 29: In Oblivion...119

Day 30: A Hope-filled Benediction...................123

Bonus: Tips for Caregivers................................127

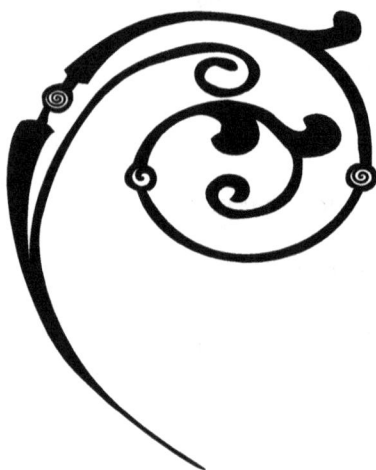

Welcome from the Author

Hello, Treasured Friend!

I wear the hats of an author, a conference speaker, a writing coach, a corporate writer for hire, a worship minister ... and more smaller roles than I can count.

But the most important of all my roles is that I'm a caregiver. It's a role that began to fall to me decades ago. One I've grown into–sometimes willingly, sometimes grudgingly. If you've picked up this book, you'll understand that better than anyone.

Thank you for joining me on this journey of being *Pressed into Care*. This book and its companion audio and eBook editions grew out of my blog, womencareforagingparents.blogspot.com.

My prayer is that this edition uplifts, encourages and re-energizes you for the sometimes long and often heart-rending task of caring for those you love as you watch them move through the stages of aging.

Each entry contains a devotional reading that's equal parts heaven's truth and earth's grit. The readings are honest about the caregiving journey.

And they're written out of my heart—in the hopes that in being transparent, I'll have the privilege of reaching your heart with the comforts and the challenges I've received along my journey—lo these many decades.

Now, then, let's get real about what happens to us when we get *Pressed Into Care* for our loved ones as they grow older.

With much prayer …
and many thoughts of blessing,

Julie Allyson

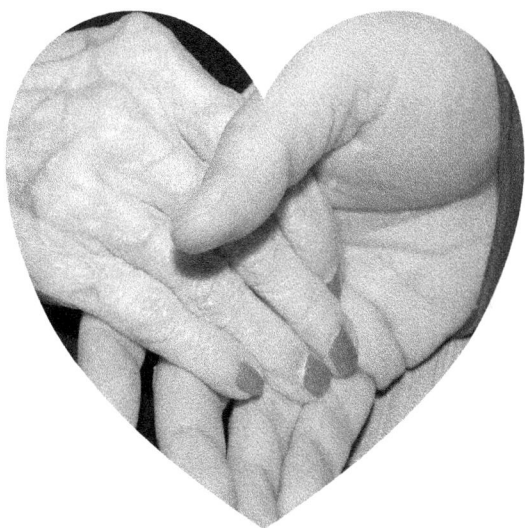

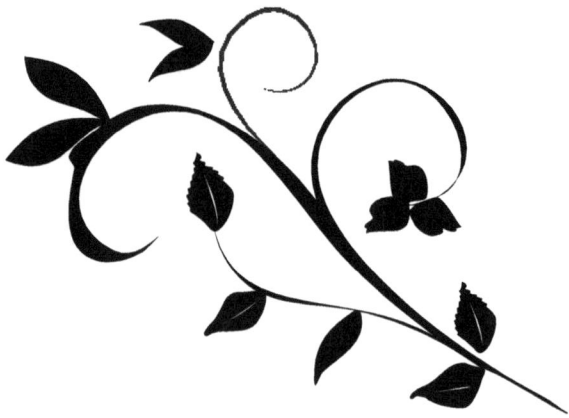

Day 1:
Treasured by God

The kingdom of heaven is like a merchant seeking fine pearls, and upon finding one pearl of great value, he went and sold all that he had and bought it (Matt. 13:45-46).

Within the last 24 hours, I had a phone call from a friend whose father was being rushed to the emergency room (she called as she was *en route* to the hospital). I also had an email from a colleague whose mother was being resettled into a nursing facility after a fall. Then I attended the memorial for one of my mother's contemporaries whose children watched her die in a long battle with cancer.

While socializing there, I cried with an acquaintance whose mother (living thousands of miles away) is tottering between life and death after having a stroke, and stood with another whose sister-in-law is in a rehab hospital. (To make matters worse, the patient's husband is in the grips of advanced dementia.)

I assured all of them that I would carry them to the Father in prayer. And I will continue to do so. But, in one very human sense, that seems so little for me to do.

As you each will attest, these crises are all too common as we watch our loved ones age. And they take a toll on us as we stand by helplessly, entrusting our precious loved ones into the care of medical teams made up, by and large, of strangers. But do our prayers really do anything for our fellow caregivers or care receivers in crisis?

So many times our lives are filled with trauma, emergency, upheaval, guilt, and distress. Perhaps that's why the Scripture I want to share with you today jumps off the page for me.

The setting is when the Prophet Daniel received a terribly unsettling revelation from the Lord. It troubled him so that he could do absolutely nothing but pour his heart out to God. He didn't eat. He didn't sleep. He didn't tend to personal hygiene. (Does that sound at all like the life of a caregiver in crisis?)

For twenty-one days this went on. (It seemed interminable, just like our heavy-duty caring times.) And then, in a moment, a messenger from heaven showed up.

Did that messenger berate Daniel for his tears? Did he tell the prophet to buck up? Did he bull right in with the discouraging diagnosis? Did he tell Daniel to stop praying and do something more productive? None of the above. Here's the way Daniel recorded what happened:

No strength was left in me; my face grew deathly pale, and I was powerless. ... Suddenly, a hand touched me and raised me to my hands and knees. He said to me, "Daniel, you are a man treasured by God. Understand the words that I'm saying to you. Stand on your feet, for I have now been sent to you." After he said this to me, I stood trembling. "Don't be afraid, Daniel," he said to me, "for from the first day that you purposed to understand and to humble yourself before your God, your prayers were heard. I have come because of your prayers" (Daniel 10:8-12, HCSB).

Three phrases jump out at me, as if they were ablaze in neon lights:

- "you are ... treasured by God"
- "don't be afraid"
- "your prayers were heard"

My friends whose parents are in crisis this day (and those of us who are in breather moments between crises), take heart. Not only does God see your exhaustion—not only does He feel your lack of strength and your powerlessness in the face of crisis, but He sends an answer—a response to your prayers.

Whatever you're facing today, know this for a fact:

- You are treasured by God.
- You don't need to remain afraid. (Think of the words of David, in Psalm 23: "I will fear no evil, for You are with me.")
- And, most of all, God hears and is even now acting on your behalf.

Treasured one, be strong and stand on your feet, for the Lord who loves you is beside you today. He was there with His servants in days past, He is with each of us today, and He will be always and forever with us.

May we find strength and encouragement from the truths of God's Word. Hearten us, Father, for today's task.

Day 2
Precious, Short-lived Solitude

"Come away by yourselves to a remote place and rest a while." For many people were coming and going, and they did not even have time to eat" (Mark 6:30-31, hcsb).

I had a single moment of solitude on one recent Saturday evening, although for a moment it didn't look like it would come to be. The place of solitude: a commuter jet heading for O'Hare Airport. It was just a quick breather, mid-weekend. I'd kissed my folks goodbye only hours before—then just as quickly I was returning home. It had been an intense 36-hour whirlwind trip, where I'd written a chapter of my Bible study book while sitting in a noisy gate area, attended a curriculum planning meeting in Colorado Springs, and was now returning home to teach an Adult Bible Fellowship and play violin in church on Sunday morning.

It was the last flight of the evening, so I expected it to be rather empty; judging from the gate area, I was right. So, I boarded early (I'd paid for the privilege) and nestled into seat 4a, folded my arms and began to doze. Suddenly my row (the three remaining seats of it) was accosted with a family of four—yes, four in three seats—little girl, dad, mom and toddler (with dirty diaper). I probably don't have to describe what was going through my mind. I fumed silently for the duration of the boarding process.

But then, bless her, the flight attendant who was about to close the aircraft door made this announcement: "Anyone who wishes may move back in the plane, where there are empty seats."

Up in a flash, I found myself the empty row 7 and sprawled across it.

Whoa! A blessing for which I was desperate. Restful moments spent with my head in my hands, praying for strength and wisdom and energy and courage and safety (for myself and for my aging parents while I was away).

I find myself in moments of solitude, rare as they are, seeking the company of my Savior. It is in His company that I, no matter how overwhelmed and exhausted, can breathe in enough heavenly oxygen to continue my heavy-laden schedule.

Jesus, thanks for the reminder that You know what I need. And sometimes that need is as basic as a moment alone with You. Would you meet that basic need today—for me and for my treasured friends who are sharing this moment with me?

Day 3
Who's With Me?

The LORD is the One who will go before you. He will be with you; He will not leave you or forsake you. Do not be afraid or discouraged" (Deut. 31:8 hcsb).

I find myself drawn to the story told in Mark chapter 6. Let me read it to you:

> The apostles gathered around Jesus and reported to Him all that they had done and taught. He said to them, "Come away by yourselves to a remote place and rest a while." For many people were coming and going, and they did not even have time to eat. So they went away in the boat by themselves to a remote place, but many saw them leaving and recognized them. People ran there by land from all the towns and arrived ahead of them (Mark 6:30-33 hcsb).

What drew my attention to this passage of Scripture from early in Jesus' ministry and to the promise from Deuteronomy that opened the chapter?

I believe we desperately need to tell our Heavenly Lord all about what's been going on in our lives. We need to lay out before Him the things that have wrung us out like the soggy sponge I left crunched up on my kitchen counter—next to the dirty dishes.

They may be good things, like those the disciples reported in Mark 6: *I've been about your ministry, Lord, and I've seen Your hand accomplish many things!* Or they may be menial or frightening or tedious things. *God, I can't take another moment of watching my loved one fade away, his mind captive to dementia, her body ravaged by disease.*

In those moments, we can be heartened by Jesus' response to the disciples—because I believe He is responding to our reports similarly today.

First, note that He didn't say *Great job. I'm impressed with all you did for Me.*

Instead, here's my paraphrase of how He did respond: *You don't even have time to eat. Let me help you take care and refresh yourself. You can't do ministry and you won't find strength for the day by heaping exhaustion upon exhaustion.*

True, the disciples' work was waiting (perhaps even multiplied) on the other side of that lake, but for a brief moment, Jesus' prescription for them was respite. I'm glad Mark doesn't give us a report about some heavy teaching Jesus gave during the trip. I suspect, if I were to imagine the scene, each disciple curled up, nibbled on his packed lunch, then cradled his neck in his pack and napped.

Like the disciples, after the food and the nap, the comfort we'll find in the Deuteronomy passage is the one that prepares us to return to the work at hand: God hasn't forsaken us or left us—and He never will. This work to which He's called me, challenging and difficult though it may be, is possible for that very reason. He calls. He's faithful. He's here with me right now. And, my treasured friend, He's right there with you, as well.

Father, please give each of us a moment of refreshment today (even in the oddest places), where we can drink in Your instruction and Your timeless promises to us.

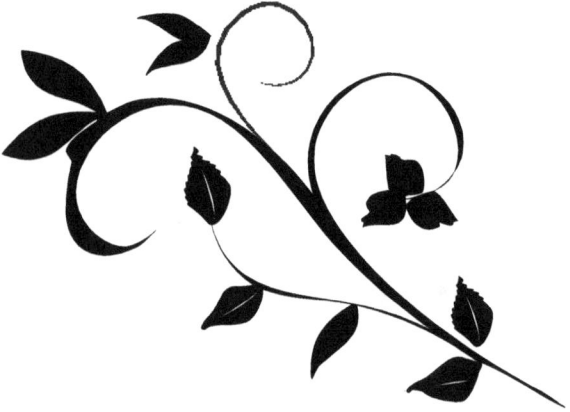

Day 4
Our Only Source of Strength

"Remain in me, and I will remain in you. No branch can bear fruit by itself; it must remain in the vine. Neither can you bear fruit unless you remain in me. I am the vine; you are the branches. If a man remains in me and I in him, he will bear much fruit; apart from me you can do nothing" (John 15:4-5).

I spent this morning teaching an adult Bible fellowship group at our church. My topic was John 15:1-10. What a beautiful and jam-packed passage that is. Our Lord, just before going to Gethsemane and then to the cross, so lovingly addressed His followers. He challenged them. He comforted them. He reminded them of all He'd been modeling before them throughout His years of ministry.

And, most relevantly for us in the midst of challenging medical situations, He had a dire yet hope-filled diagnosis for how our lives will be measured, from His vantage point. Here's the striking revelation: unless we remain in Him, we can do *nothing*!

Faithful caregiver, exhausted patient, in the drudgery and life-sapping tasks, you probably have no problem with the concept that your strength isn't sufficient for the day. I know there have been many days, humanly speaking, when the demands on me far surpass my energy stores. You may be living one of those today.

But Jesus didn't tell us that we *couldn't do much* apart from being connected to Him. He didn't say, there are some things that you'll need *a little help* doing. He didn't say, sometimes you'll want to plug into me for a little extra something. No! He said, "Without me, your best efforts will amount to nothing."

Nothing? Really, Jesus? I'm doing so many things because it's right for me to do them. Okay, so sometimes, I forget to get recharged or to ask for Your direction. But it all counts for nothing? That's a drastic diagnosis to give me when I'm trying so hard!

Pretty discouraging stuff, if He'd left it there. But the good news is that there's more to the story—in fact, He gave us the good news ahead of the bad news. Let's look again at verse 5, this time from the NLT, because there it really pops:

> "Yes, I am the vine; you are the branches. Those who remain in me, and I in them, will produce much fruit. For apart from me you can do nothing."

In Christ, *through* Christ, and *by* Christ, our labors will be more productive than we could ever imagine. They will bear "much fruit." Not a little. But a lot of juicy, fruity, nourishing sweetness will come bursting out of our lives. That's what I want to be a part of producing, don't you?

What does this fruit look like in real life? In our prayer time in ABF this morning, we heard about a man who is battling cancer. He's a man of strong faith in Christ. And, as we were going to prayer on his behalf, we heard this report: his wife says her faith has been strengthened as she's watched him and cared for him through the illness that has him in its grasp. This brother in Christ is *remaining*—he is showing by a life well lived that not through human effort, but through Christ's life shining through his suffering, his branch is bearing fruit for the kingdom of God.

So, the challenge to each of us today is clear. Remain attached to the vine of Christ. It's not an option, not one thing among many to drop down the rungs of our to-do lists until we get more time. It's crucial—it's life-giving—and it makes all the difference in the world.

Father, may we remain attached to Christ today—and in our remaining, may He bear much fruit through our lives as we give ourselves away in care for those we love and as we battle the illnesses that are threatening to get us down.

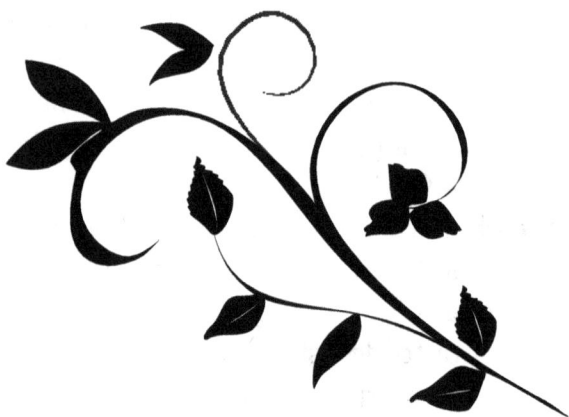

Day 5
A Gethsemane Request

Then Jesus came with them to a place called Gethsemane, and said to His disciples, "Sit here while I go over there and pray." And He took with Him Peter and the two sons of Zebedee, and began to be grieved and distressed. Then He said to them, "My soul is deeply grieved, to the point of death; remain here and keep watch with Me" (Matt. 26:36-38).

As I write, I'm remembering Christ's passion for us, and I'm spending some time contemplating and examining Matthew's eyewitness account of the last hours before Jesus was arrested, tried, convicted, and crucified.

In particular, I'm drawn anew to the moments He spent praying in Gethsemane. When I read the Scripture that opened this entry, here's what jumped out to me.

The *grieved* and *distressed*, these I understand. As my pastor pointed out this morning—this grief, this distress that Jesus experienced in that hour and the much greater suffering in the hours that followed—those He experienced on my behalf, and yours. No one on this planet or in all of creation could take His place or do what He was called on to do in that hour. Only He could carry our sins, our grief, our sorrows, our pain. There was no other alternative. If we were to be rescued from the curse of Eden's sin, only Christ could enter into death itself to buy us back at the cost of His precious lifeblood.

But this simple request of our Master as He faced the hour that would culminate in the reason He entered space and time in human form, is so telling. "I'm in distress, my friends, and I need you to just be here with me in this moment." There was nothing the disciples could do to lessen Christ's load. He would never permit it.

(Remember the conversation, probably just weeks before, when Peter blurted out the claim that he never would let his Master be put to death? Jesus had a quick and strong rebuke for His friend—"Get behind Me, Satan! You are a stumbling block to Me; for you are not setting your mind on God's interests, but man's" [Matt. 16:23]).

No, there was no way anyone could lessen the Messiah's suffering—except simply by *being* with Him in this hour. Much like Mary who had anointed Jesus' feet with costly perfume days earlier in Bethany, these three inner-circle friends (Peter included) had the opportunity to sit with Jesus as He poured out His grief and distress to the Father.

If you know the rest of the story, you know the disciples weren't up to the task, for exhaustion (and perhaps grief) overtook them. But the significance here is that even Christ, in this moment of high drama and overwhelming intensity, called on trusted loved ones to sit beside Him.

Which brings us to the significance of this passage to us as we face illnesses of various kinds: The beauty of being members of Christ's family is that in compassion, camaraderie, and comfort, we can just *be* with each other in our most challenging and grievous moments. No one can be the daughter to my parents except me. No one can perform your role in your loved one's life, either. But we can stand together (or sit together) to pour out our hearts and share our stories and remind each other that we're not alone. We are a family, and when one hurts we all close ranks to offer hearts of compassion and ears to listen and arms to hug and eyes to share tears.

I have the privilege of being part of a prayer team—a team of caregivers across several states— all of whom read *The Overwhelmed Woman's Guide to … Caring for Aging Parents* and decided they needed each other's prayer support as they went about the challenging tasks of honoring their aging parents. When I heard about the group, I asked if I could be a part of it. I can't tell you what a blessing these women are to me—in fact we drove an hour each to be together just this weekend. We have the opportunity, via cyberspace and occasionally in person, to just be with each other in these deeply grievous times.

But there is even better news yet … the God/Man Christ experienced in that hour in the

Garden of Gethsemane my grief—and yours. He knows how it feels. He knew what it meant to be overwhelmed with sorrow to the point of distress and exhaustion. He experienced it all for us—and He will sit with us in our moments today, if we will but drop our pack of burdens before Him in honest, heartfelt prayer.

Father, I thank you that I don't even need Internet access to get to You—and You won't ever fall asleep when I ask you to be near me. I am grateful to know You watch and pray with me.

Day 6
Christ's Passion for
Our Saddest Times

He was despised and rejected by men, a man of suffering who knew what sickness was. He was like someone people turned away from; He was despised, and we didn't value Him (Isa. 53:6).

In my study these days, I've been turning my attention to the way God revealed Christ's passion to the prophet Isaiah centuries before Jesus' birth. It's a familiar passage in Isaiah 53, but one I believe has special relevance to us as caregivers—who daily work to assuage another's pains, all the while battling our own griefs, sorrows, disappointments, agonies, and illnesses.

Listen, weary caregiver, to how closely Jesus identified with your circumstances while His body was being torn to shreds by the stripes, while His lifeblood was spattering down, while He was gasping for each fleeting breath.

I'll use the HCSB translation, which may sound a little different from the one you've heard or read most often. (I do this intentionally, because sometimes reading the same truth with a different cadence arrests our attention and envelopes us in old truth from a new perspective.)

> He was despised and rejected by men, a man of suffering who knew what sickness was. He was like someone people turned away from; He was despised, and we didn't value Him.
>
> Yet He Himself bore our sicknesses, and He carried our pains; but we in turn regarded Him stricken, struck down by God, and afflicted.
>
> But He was pierced because of our transgressions, crushed because of our iniquities; punishment for our peace was on Him, and we are healed by His wounds.
>
> We all went astray like sheep; we all have turned to our own way; and the LORD has punished Him for the iniquity of us all. (Isa. 53:3-6, HCSB)

When my pastor preached on this passage not long ago, he keyed in on the fact that as Isaiah prophesied this event, he mentioned our sicknesses and pains early on. This is significant, he said, letting us see how closely Jesus identified with us at our weakest points of human suffering. He knew what sickness was!

As He took the stripes and felt the nails tear into His flesh:

- He felt the exhaustion of every home-tied caregiver whose back aches from lifting her parent from bed to wheelchair.

- He felt the shredding sorrow of the long goodbye dementia patients and their loved ones endure.

- He felt the grief of death's separation.

- He felt the uncertainty you're experiencing as you're doing your best for your parent but you fear your best may not be nearly enough.

He felt it, He bore it, and He offers hope through His resurrection that in His completion of the transaction through His death and resurrection, there will be a day when we will know what is already known in the realms of Eternity ... sorrow, sighing, tears, and pain have all been swept away by the flow of His precious blood down that awful cross and into the desert sands outside Jerusalem that day.

Yes, have all been swept away. What we're experiencing here, though it feels so permanent, so real, so absolutely endless, is more like an evaporating vapor than a concrete reality, at least from Heaven's perspective. Through the prophet God speaks what will be as if it already had been— by His stripes, we are healed.

So, as we go about our day of pain, rehab, illness, or caregiving my prayer is that each of us will try on this Heavenly reality for size—not only is Christ side-by-side with us in our most grievous tasks, but He has already conquered them for every believer who trusts in Him for ultimate and complete salvation.

God, give me comfort and strength for today's challenges, drawing on the resources from Jesus bearing my pain in His body on the cross.

Day 7
He Is Risen!

He will swallow up death for all time,
And the Lord GOD will wipe tears away from all faces
(Isa. 25:8).

We all experience days that make us appreciate good friends, stable health, and time together as a family. There were six of us around the Easter supper table on one of those especially poignant days: my parents and I were joined by our dear friends—two adult daughters and their widowed mom. Despite all of us having endured innumerable trips to surgeons, doctors, test facilities, pharmacies, emergency rooms, and rehab facilities, on that day we were all together and for the moment on the better side, health-wise.

We around the table had been through our seasons of such intense illness that a holiday meal together was unthinkable. That probably made the day all that much sweeter for the six of us—reflecting on how God brought us through stormy seasons, reflecting on our loved ones who were already absent from the body and present with the Lord; reflecting on the hope that keeps us going when the weeks again become Everest-like treks devoid of Sherpa guides.

Our shared meal was a reminder for me that we all need continuous encouragement that comes from the reminder that seasons pass. Our days won't always be sunny, yet our load won't always be unbearable. The hope of Easter is exactly that. *There will be a day when ...*

> The LORD of hosts will prepare a lavish banquet for all peoples ... He will swallow up death for all time, And the Lord GOD will wipe tears away from all faces, And He will remove the reproach of His people from all the earth; For the LORD has spoken. And it will be said in that day, "Behold, this is our God for whom we have waited that He might save us. This is the LORD for whom we have waited; Let us rejoice and be glad in His salvation" (Isa. 25:6-9).

Imagine what that celebration will be like. Heavenly chefs placing before a gathering of saints from all nations and all generations the most lavish and bountiful spread ever tabled. And the Lord of love and grace—the Savior of Resurrection Sunday—presiding at the head as Master of the Household of Faith. Before the meal, He will come to each one and with His own nail-pierced hand brush away all tears, removing, as He does this, the last residue of sorrow and mourning and pain and suffering from our sojourn on fallen earth. With that, the joy of salvation will erupt in a magnitude never before expressed.

Looking toward this day can become our motivator—our hope—our assurance—as a season of illness or caregiving looms ahead of us. All this is possible, because it is Jesus' expressed desire: "I want them to be with Me where I am." On the night before His crucifixion Christ told the Father. "I want them to see My glory, the glory I had before the foundation of the world" (from John 17).

That's why there was a cross for Christ. That's why there was a crown of thorns twisted into His brow and a spear in His side and a burial shroud draped across His battered earthly shell.

That's why there was a boulder rolled across the entrance of a borrowed tomb by hulking Roman soldiers.

That's why it took two angels in white robes to break the seal and an earthquake to roll away the hunk of solid earth and sit atop it—readying the grand announcement:

He is not here.
He is risen, as He said.

Sure the amazing news of the Resurrection stunned even His inner circle. They'd stood by helplessly—as if in the most horrid nightmare— while their Master was cruelly and brutally massacred by a crowd of easily swayed countrymen and foreigner soldiers. But with Christ's resurrection in the power of the Holy Spirit (Rom. 1:4), death would no longer win—it would never be the end for those who believe in Him. The cruelest suffering on earth will pale in that day when it's wiped away by the loving hand of our Lord. All that will remain will be our knowledge of His faithfulness, His love, His grace, His mercy—and our undying gratitude for it.

Take hope, my friend. No matter what you're facing today, let the empty tomb be your eternal reminder that Christ didn't just experience your griefs beside you, didn't just carry them with you, but He conquered them once for all time for you. The tomb is empty, so your exhaustion and your suffering do not have the last word. He has conquered, and He will one day allow you to see that the spoils of His victory belong to you.

Father, God, may the truth of the Resurrection of Jesus Christ be my strength today.

Day 8
No Better Helper

*But if we hope for what we do not yet have, we wait for it
patiently. In the same way, the Spirit helps us in our
weakness. We do not know what we ought to pray for, but
the Spirit himself intercedes for us with groans that words
cannot express. And he who searches our hearts knows the
mind of the Spirit, because the Spirit intercedes for the saints
in accordance with God's will (Rom. 8:25-27).*

One of the places in the Word where I go for
comfort early and often is Romans 8. This whole
chapter overflows with such beauty—such
assurance. In its truths I've found resources I never
knew I could tap.

For example, verse 21 assures us that we, along
with all creation—and especially our ailing loved
ones—will be liberated one day from our bondage
to decay. The aging process will one day be
conquered by perfect health. Death will be
overcome by life, rather than the other way around.

Even if we sometimes watch as decay takes the
upper hand, what a comfort to have the absolute
assurance that what we see isn't the last word—
Someone else has the last word, the Someone
whose Father didn't allow His body to decay in the

grave, the Someone who rose and conquered death itself, the Someone Who now holds in His nail-scarred hands the keys of death, hell and the grave.

This is such a rich passage for us, that I'd like us to focus on a couple more truths from its verses.

Today, let's look at our source of strength and comfort as we give ourselves away in caring for our aging loved ones. I quoted it earlier in Romans 8:25-27.

Did you catch the phrase as I read, "the Spirit helps us in our weakness"? The Spirit of God, Third Person of the Trinity, that Spirit—Comforter, Counselor, Friend—He recognizes our weakness, our exhaustion, our pain, our discouragement. And not only that, He comes in, rolls up His sleeves (as it were), gets into the middle of our struggles, and helps us. The HCSB translation puts it this way: "the Spirit also joins to help in our weakness." *NASB Greek Dictionary* clarifies the long, compound Greek word Paul used when he wrote this. "To take hold with at the side, … to take a share in, generally to help."

So, treasured friend, today you need not feel alone. If there were only One Who could ever be on your side, at your side, shouldering the weight of the load along with you—you would want it to be this One—the Spirit of the Living God. Who better to search our hearts and help us in our most trying moments?

Next time we'll focus on His prayers for us. But for today, let's bask in the knowledge that His place is right where we are—right in the middle of it all—and He's lending His more than sufficient aid on our behalf.

God, I draw strength in this moment from the promise that the Spirit is helping me in my weakest hours. This is my hope—founded on solid ground. I choose to take comfort from it.

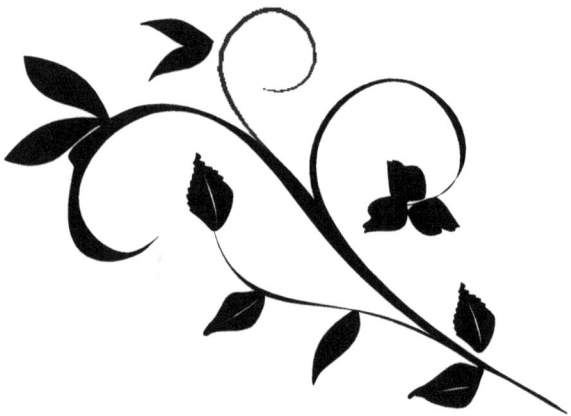

Day 9
So Very Close

We do not know what we ought to pray for, but the Spirit himself intercedes for us with groans that words cannot express (Rom. 8:26).

One of the easiest necessities to let slide amid flurries of medical diagnoses, financial concerns, and legal issues—is the element of spending love-filled quality time with our families and nearest friends. And yet what we need most of all is sweet time enjoying the companionship of those with whom we've built relationships over the course of lifetimes.

As I plan to do with my mom today, I challenge you to just sit with your loved one, listen to her, talk about something other than illness or disabilities. Just be together. I have a friend who does this, and for her it's most difficult. Her mom is in the throes of dementia and has stopped talking or even responding most days. Yet, my friend goes to sit with her mom, every week, just to chat. A one-sided conversation, to be sure. A monologue. Yet she chatters on. Telling her mom news from the world outside the nursing facility's walls. News of children and grandchildren, friends and church. Not expecting or needing a response. But simply sharing her heart, in the hopes that it will reach her mom somewhere in her mind's prison.

This is a concept I believe translates well into our relationship with God and our dependence on His Spirit as we go about our lives. Listen to the closeness of relationship Paul describes regarding the believer and the Spirit of God Who lives within us:

> In the same way, the Spirit helps us in our weakness. We do not know what we ought to pray for, but the Spirit himself intercedes for us with groans that words cannot express.

> And he who searches our hearts knows the mind of the Spirit, because the Spirit intercedes for the saints in accordance with God's will (Rom. 8:26-27).

He's so close that He searches our hearts. We don't even need to form words to let Him know our needs, our exhaustion, our desperation, our utter dependence. He searches our hearts and recognizes our needs at the deepest levels. And He's the same one Who knows the heart of our loving Father toward us. So, He asks the Father for what we need most—and He does this in line with what He already knows to be the Father's perfect will for us. And don't think for a moment that our Father in

Heaven won't answer His own Spirit's intercessory requests on our behalf with a resounding "Yes! Amen! Let it be done!"

This is quality relationship at its most amazing. The Triune God knows us. He is in us and with us and works through us. And, as we'll discover soon (in Romans 8:38-39) His love for us is beyond deterioration, division, or distraction. Nothing—not even the most grievous parts of the aging process— can separate us from His love, demonstrated most clearly in the gift of Christ Jesus our Lord.

Father, God, help me today to spend quality time with my loved ones. More importantly help me spend quality time getting to know You, Who knows me so intimately.

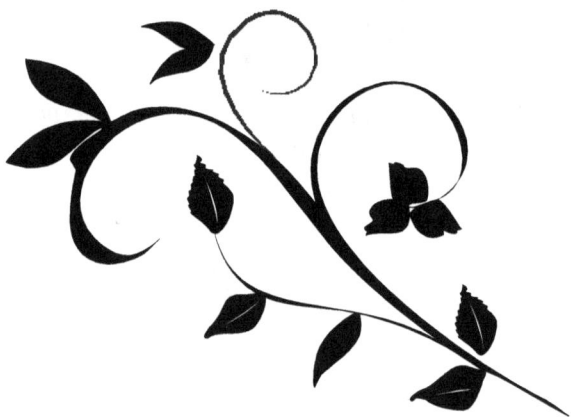

Day 10

Overwhelmed!

We are more than victorious through Him who loved us (Rom. 8:37).

This week I've been in special prayer for two dear fellow-caregivers who are making the agonizing decisions about the best facilities where their ailing parents will get the care they desperately need. To make these choices in their parents' best interests, these loving caregivers need more wisdom, insight, calm, compassion, strength, tenacity, and assistance than they can get in human terms. But, as both are also long-time followers of Christ, they have the assurance that they are not alone, that through prayer and listening for God's direction they will find the resources they need so desperately.

The best news is that you, too, can have that same assurance.

Listen to the words Paul penned to bolster fellow sufferers in their times of most stringent battle:

Who can separate us from the love of Christ? Can affliction or anguish or persecution or famine or nakedness or danger or sword? As it is written: Because of You we are being put to death all day long; we are counted as sheep to be slaughtered.

No, in all these things we are more than victorious through Him who loved us.

For I am persuaded that not even death or life, angels or rulers, things present or things to come, hostile powers, height or depth, or any other created thing will have the power to separate us from the love of God that is in Christ Jesus our Lord! (Rom. 8:35-39, HCSB).

Not even death—not even people or circumstances—not even illness or pain or grief—none of these things and nothing anywhere can separate us from the love of God. Drink in that awesome truth.

I've often wondered why Paul keyed in on the love attribute of God here. Why not, nothing can separate us from the power of God? or the wisdom of God? or the deliverance of God? While those are all true, there's something special about the agape love of God—the love that gives itself away for the betterment of the beloved. The love that puts the needs of another ahead of its own comfort. That's the perfect and complete love from which nothing—

not even the darkest day of caregiving—can ever separate us.

God the victor. God the destroyer of death, hell, and the grave. God the wise. God the all-powerful. Not only does He hold all these titles. But He holds them for our lives—all wrapped up in the package of His love. How much more comforting is it that the One Who is so mighty chooses to use that might on our behalf, in love, with our best interests (and those of our loved ones) in His heart of hearts?

So, fatigued and overwhelmed friend, draw courage and strength from the amazing love of God for you.

Yes, life is tragically difficult at times. But the One Who loves you perfectly is connected to you, next to you, yoked to you inseparably. He is pulling with you, and no one can change that.

Maybe your definition of "victorious through Him who loves you" doesn't look exactly like you thought it would today. But you can come through stronger and closer to Him and more convinced of His love for you today than you were yesterday. And maybe that's not such a bad tradeoff.

God, I love the sound of this promise: that I can be victorious through You, because You love me. I choose to bask in Your victory.

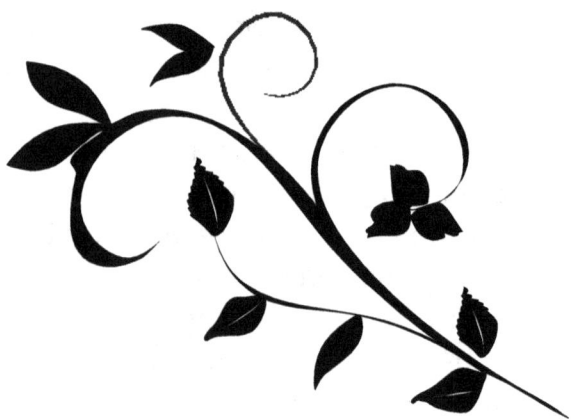

Day 11
Cling to This

Let us not lose heart in doing good (Gal. 6:9).

I've been feeling spiritually wrung out these days. Chasing to doctor visits. Worried and concerned about many things—like Martha (Luke 10:41). Missing out on the truly important, I've resisted the opportunity to use these moments of testing in my life to draw closer in my relationship with Christ.

Perhaps you've been through some seasons like this, as well.

As I was praying this morning, confessing that I simply didn't feel like having a quiet time with the Lord, the words of this long-ago memorized passage came to mind—and in them I found a measure of strength and energy to press on:

> Let us not lose heart in doing good, for in due time we will reap if we do not grow weary. So then, while we have opportunity, let us do good to all people, and especially to those who are of the household of the faith (Gal. 6:9-10).

It seems the Apostle Paul recognized in the Galatian believers (probably from having experienced the same temptation himself) fatigue— a drained-to-the-dregs feeling that had them sure none of the effort they were spending would ultimately prove worthwhile.

His prescription was to press on through—keep doing good and keep your heart in it. There will be a dividend one day, even if you can't see it right now. Don't be weary. (That sounds a lot like the Master's words in John 14:1, "Don't let your heart be troubled. Trust Me.")

It seems to me the second half of the prescription is to find and seize every opportunity to keep doing good—to everyone. Does that include the doctor who may not be treating my loved one with the tender care as if he were his own flesh and blood? Does that include the client who is delinquent in paying what is owed? Does that include the driver who cuts me off on the road? Or the customer service agent who seems more interested in venting her own frustration than in helping solve my problem with her company?

I suppose the "everyone" in the passage includes all those individuals—and so many more. And especially those in the household (whether God's household or our own). Those closest. Those most likely to hear our tirades. Those who need our "doing good" the most.

I'm not quite sure how this works, exactly. Because Paul (and Christ) tell us simply not to let it happen. The weariness. The discouragement. The feeling that none of this battle is worth the effort. They make it sound like a choice—a change in perspective. And perhaps it is. Looking toward another eventuality—the one that is in what seems like the far distant future (but could be as close as this very hour). In light of eternity this "momentary light affliction is producing for us an absolutely incomparable eternal weight of glory" (2 Cor. 4:17, HCSB).

God, I'm weary. I need You to sustain me today. May I sense the eternal glory even in this affliction that doesn't seem so light or momentary to me. I choose to cling to Your Word, no matter how I feel.

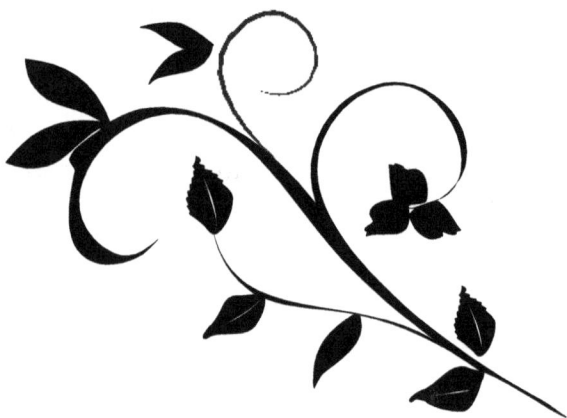

Day 12
Hide and Seek

He who has my laws and keeps them, he it is who has love for me: and he who has love for me will be loved by my Father, and I will have love for him and will let myself be seen clearly by him (John 14:21 BBE).

One of my favorite Daddy times was in our old house, when I was a tiny tot. Daddy commuted downtown, so he was gone thirteen exhausting hours every day. But he was just a very tall little boy, at heart. He loved to play. So, no matter how weary he felt, he always was up for a game of hide and seek while Mom finished preparing supper.

Daddy was creative in his hiding places. It took me lots of giggles, restarts, and slammed closet doors before he'd jump out of his hiding place and scare me. More giggles. When I'd hide, though, odds were better than 50/50 I'd be behind the bathtub curtain. My goal, you see, wasn't so much to hide, as to be found. My game was about the tickles, hugs and laughter of being lifted into Daddy's arms.

This memory flooded my mind today. How different these memories are from my last memories of Daddy. We'd exchanged roles somewhere along the way. In those later years, amid the shots and meds and balanced meals I helped him with, what meant the most to him were the moments I paid attention to his stories—yes again!—giggling and hugging and making him feel the way he had made me feel all those years ago: Important. Special. Loved. Those were painful days in the end, but now that they're over, I've never been sorry I made time to show him love.

With all these musings, my Scripture reading led me to John 14: 21 where Jesus promised to those who love and obey Him the greatest gift of all: He'll reveal Himself to us. The Greek word could be translated as "disclose." He's not playing hide and seek with us–but the minute we seek Him, He begins to unfold to us His amazing grace and mercy, not to mention His magnificent, holy presence.

This perplexed the disciples, because Jude asked, "How is it that you will let yourself be seen clearly by us and not by the world?" (v. 22). Why do we get to see You, but the world doesn't? Why don't You show Your power and establish Your global reign right now?

Jesus had a ready answer: "If anyone has love for me, he will keep my words: and he will be dear to my Father; and we will come to him and make our living-place with him." (v. 23).

Just like my moment of being lifted into Daddy's arms, our Heavenly Father longs to lift His loving children into His mighty, compassionate arms. He loves us. And He's waiting only for us to love and seek Him. When we do, an amazing relationship of unspeakable joy awaits.

Heavenly Father, help me to love as You love. Help me to value my aging loved one as You do. Give me the tender heart to take the time to show them love even when the days get so long and demanding. Amen.

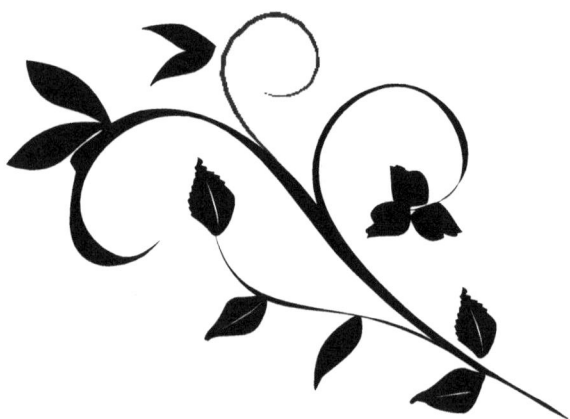

Day 13
When the Well Is Dry

May the LORD answer you in the day of trouble! May the name of the God of Jacob set you securely on high! May He send you help from the sanctuary! (Psa. 20:1).

Recently, we asked our circle to pray for us, because we were facing impending surgery, work challenges (life does go on!), and more.

So, for me, the well seems dry. That's why I returned one evening to a Scripture my grandfather bequeathed to me in a card shortly before his death. I've found it meaningful as I've read it over and over in the last thirty years. That night, I confess, it made me cry—the good kind of tears.

I pray it will touch your heart in much the same way—at your point of most humbling need.

> May the LORD answer you in the day of trouble!
> May the name of the God of Jacob set you securely on high!
> May He send you help from the sanctuary
> And support you from Zion!
> May He remember all your meal offerings
> And find your burnt offering acceptable! Selah.
> May He grant you your heart's desire

And fulfill all your counsel!
We will sing for joy over your victory,
And in the name of our God we will set up our
banners.
May the LORD fulfill all your petitions.
Now I know that the LORD saves His anointed;
He will answer him from His holy heaven With
the saving strength of His right hand.
Some boast in chariots and some in horses,
But we will boast in the name of the LORD, our
God (Psa. 20:1-7).

The strength in this passage, for me, is not just the confidence in God's strength, but the fact that a cheerleader out there somewhere is carrying me to the throne of God even this moment. I know this because the Bible tells us that there are two Heavenly Prayer Warriors constantly speaking my name and yours to the Father—Jesus Christ and the Holy Spirit. And, joining Their voices, in this passage, are godly friends—all pulling in the same direction, asking God to strengthen us and to prove Himself faithful to us.

Let's make a covenant ... you and I ... I'm praying this passage for you as I write tonight—and please pray it for me whenever you read it. I'm quite sure I'll need it! As will you.

God, I pray for others who are suffering today. Will You answer them in their distress even as You answer me in mine?

Day 14
Here We Go Again!

But now thus says the LORD ... "When you pass through the waters, I will be with you; and through the rivers, they shall not overwhelm you ... you are precious in my eyes" (Isa. 43:1-4; ESV).

This week we've spent more time than we'd hoped in hospital waiting rooms (you'd recognize the antiseptic smell anywhere, and you won't soon forget the uniquely metallic chill common to the exam rooms). And it's not going to get easier any time soon.

You know how that goes—because you've been there (or perhaps are there), too.

That's why this Scripture promise from the mouth of God has been extra meaningful to me this week:

But now thus says the LORD, he who created you, O Jacob, he who formed you, O Israel: "Fear not, for I have redeemed you; I have called you by name, you are mine. When you pass through the waters, I will be with you; and through the rivers, they shall not overwhelm you; when you walk through fire you shall not

be burned, and the flame shall not consume
you.
For I am the LORD your God, the Holy One of
Israel, your Savior " (Isa. 43:1-3; ESV).

I really don't like that one word that keeps
cropping up in the passage: when. God doesn't say,
if the waters threaten to flood you out; if you find
yourself walking through fire or if flames come
close to you. It's that pesky when. These things do
come close to us—they do touch our households,
our loved ones, our own bodies. It's a reality and a
certainty—it's going to happen. The question is
how we're going to make it through.

For followers of Christ, the comfort is in the
companionship. It is in *Who* has called us by name,
Who wades into the waters and *Who* walks
alongside us to keep our feet from sliding on mossy
rocks, Who knows where the invisible sand pits cut
into the slimy river bed, and Who pledges to keep
us from falling into them.

Like He did for the three Hebrew youths in the
king's triple-hot furnace, Christ Himself will be for
us the fourth man right in there with us keeping the
fire's flames from kindling on us. I love that scene,
told in Daniel 3. Because, although God allowed the
fires near His faithful followers, when (I like this use
of when much better!) He brought them out of the
furnace, their clothes weren't even singed—they
didn't even have the smell of smoke lingering in
their hair. Their faith rings in my ears:

"Our God whom we serve is able to deliver us from the furnace of blazing fire; and He will deliver us out of your hand, O king. But even if He does not, let it be known to you, O king, that we are not going to serve your gods or worship the golden image that you have set up" (Dan. 3:17-18).

The similarity between Daniel 3's action and Isaiah 43's promise brings me comfort in the assurance that God will again be true to His Word—*Fear not! ... I will be with you.* He has the means to follow through on His promise, and the inclination (because He loves us and because He formed us and called us His own) to do so.

God, what You say, You will do. I cling to this assurance even when the flood of caregiving and fires of uncertainty threaten to overwhelm me.

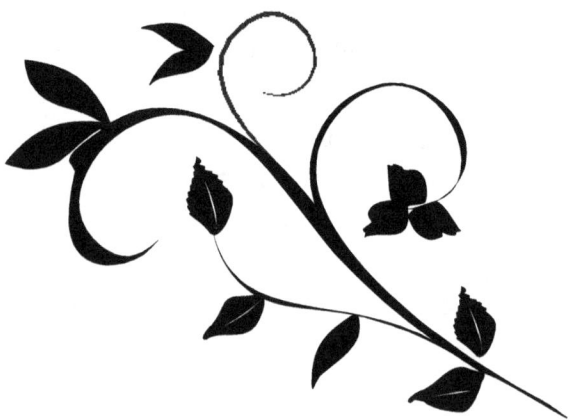

Day 15
Answered Prayer

The eyes of the LORD are toward the righteous And His ears are open to their cry (Psa. 34:15).

I want to offer you a glimpse into how the Lord intervened on our family's behalf on one special occasion—clearly and obviously—and beyond what we expected. First, let me share a portion of the Scripture our pastors Greg and Tim read to Dad (and us) in his hospital room that morning. It's from Psalm 34. When you have time, read the whole Psalm—for it is a faith-builder. But here's a portion of it that rang true for us:

> Psalm 34:1-15 (NASB)
> I will bless the LORD at all times; His praise shall continually be in my mouth.
>
> My soul will make its boast in the LORD; The humble will hear it and rejoice. O magnify the LORD with me, And let us exalt His name together. I sought the LORD, and He answered me, And delivered me from all my fears. They looked to Him and were radiant, And their faces will never be ashamed. This poor man cried,

and the LORD heard him And saved him out of all his troubles. The angel of the LORD encamps around those who fear Him, And rescues them.

O taste and see that the LORD is good; How blessed is the man who takes refuge in Him! ... The eyes of the LORD are toward the righteous And His ears are open to their cry.

And here's what the Lord did for Dad a few hours later ... as I reported it to my email prayer team:

You're really not going to believe this one ... We got to the hospital, went through all the admission, pre-op, our pastors came and prayed with us, and the nurse brought him down for the procedure. They hooked up IV, and put him on the pacemaker monitor and .... his heart had corrected on its own. No procedure!

They came and got Mom and me in the waiting room (I'd read exactly two pages of my book) and sent the three of us on our way.

What an answered prayer! I mean no disrespect to our faith here, but we simply can't believe how God undertook in answer to prayer.

I have no problem expecting God to heal through doctors and medicines, but I'm sure I didn't have the faith to even ask that He'd intervene on His own without the procedure on that morning.

Sadly, it doesn't always happen this way. In fact, we didn't know at the time that there would be a day that ended far differently. But on that day, God had in store for us one of His special surprises.

I pray today that God will be with you on your journey and show you the surprise of His hand evident and at work in your situation.

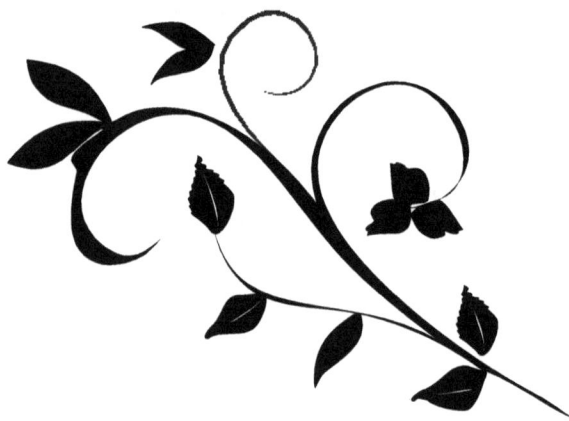

Day 16
A Degree I Don't Want

I'm pretty sure I qualified for an honorary degree courtesy of walking with Dad through his recent medical odyssey. I've secretly aspired to one for years. Not that I don't appreciate the black robe, and red and white hood I earned for my MA all those years ago at Ball State. I do. I worked hard for it—anyone who's earned one knows they're not simply bestowed, they indicate years of effort.

But as much as I've wished for an honorary degree I haven't technically earned, I'm thinking the one I qualified for after a recent trial may not be one I ought to wear with pride. It's a Ph.W.D.—you may have earned one too, a Doctorate of the Philosophy of Worries. In my waiting-room hours and especially the long nights when I lay awake imagining the absolute worst eventualities, I'm quite sure I took the study of this particular science to new heights. Oh how I've worried, fretted, fidgeted, and feared.

And it's begun taking its toll. Since I've been living it, I haven't been as conscious of its escalation—or of all the energies I've been pouring into this study. But, recently we ran into a nurse who cared for Dad in one of his earlier hospitalizations. We've seen her frequently in the ensuing years—and she's offered a listening ear and wise counsel more times than we could count. But when we saw her this time, she looked Mom and me in the eye. "This has taken its toll on you. All this worry. All this stress. You're feeling it, aren't you?"

Mom and I looked at each other. She knows our little secret. She can see in our drawn faces: the color of strain. The tell-tale lines of sleepless nights. The slump of pent-up fatigue. We nodded dumbly—and changed the subject expertly. But I couldn't get that conversation out of my mind as I tried to settle my thoughts, calm my upset gut, and un-kink my shoulder muscles in preparation for bedtime.

Something about her concern and her candor reminded me of words our Master just might have said to us in that store aisle today, had He been visibly present:

> And which of you by being anxious can add a single hour to his span of life? ... Consider the lilies of the field, how they grow: they neither toil nor spin, yet I tell you, even Solomon in all his glory was not arrayed like one of these. But if God so clothes the grass of the field, which today is alive and tomorrow is thrown into the oven, will he not much more clothe you, O you of little faith? Therefore do not be anxious,

saying, 'What shall we eat?' or 'What shall we drink?' or 'What shall we wear?' For the Gentiles seek after all these things, and your heavenly Father knows that you need them all. But seek first the kingdom of God and his righteousness, and all these things will be added to you. Therefore do not be anxious about tomorrow, for tomorrow will be anxious for itself. Sufficient for the day is its own trouble (Matthew 6:27-34; ESV).

Gospel writer Matthew records five instances where Jesus chides His devoted but weary and worried followers for their "little faith." (Matt. 6, 8:26, 14:31, 16:8, 17:20). I looked them up. And for some reason, tonight when I read them again, I wasn't my usual self—quick to wag my index finger at the disciples. This time, I understood. More than I ever have before, I resonated with the slowness of the disciples to trust the Master when circumstances look hopeless:

> • The boat is tossed by relentless winds—
> and the infuriatingly unconcerned Master
> sleeps in the bow.
> • Peter steps out of the boat and sinks into
> the waves.
> • The ministry team's tangible reserves of
> life's necessities are depleted.
> • The cure they pray for is slow in coming.

I get where they were finding their fears. Because I'm there. Right there. Worried, not that the Master can't intervene. But rather that He won't. After all, in this life, things don't always work out with fairy tale endings. Even those who received miracles in the New Testament, eventually passed out of this world and into eternity. Nothing this side is permanent. So it's easy to worry about that—to look around at circumstances, and waver in my faith. (I'm saying *my* here, but I'm guessing *you've* been here, too.)

That's where Jesus' words in Matthew 6 both challenge and encourage us. Once we get past His nailing me for my little faith and nod in agreement with His realistic assessment that "tomorrow will be anxious for itself" (it will certainly have its share of trouble), we can sink our weary selves into the middle of the passage. Usually, when I read it, I focus on the seeking first His kingdom. Certainly that's the prescription—ultimately. But tonight, I gravitated more to the "why" we needn't worry. *Abba* Father in Heaven knows what's happening here. He knows what we need. His arm is ready to act on our behalf—maybe to deliver us from the storm, more likely to support and provide for us through it. He promised He would indeed see to our needs.

So, I believe if He were to be the one to endow me with that honorary doctorate, it wouldn't be in a joyfully pleasant ceremony. I would look into His eyes and find in them a reflection of my lacking faith. I imagine He would say close to what He told the disciples on those many occasions: "Oh you of little faith, why did you doubt? Didn't you know I care? I love you? I'll add to you all the things I already know you need today—and all those things I know you'll need tomorrow. Your worry is accomplishing nothing—in fact, less than nothing. It's hurting you. It's something I don't want for you. You didn't need to earn this particular degree. Cease striving, and rest like your Master in the bow of the rocking boat. Your Mighty God has it all under control."

On second thought, maybe I'll turn down that degree, and see if I can *earn* one in a more appropriate field—I think I'll go for a P.F.D.—a Doctorate of Practical Faith. As long as it's well-placed faith in this loving and compassionate Master, it will be worth the work. Want to join me in the preparation and study?

God of all comfort , we ask that You will sustain, encourage, uplift, and strengthen our bodies, minds, and spirits. May You touch our souls with glimpses of the eternal glory that awaits us in Christ Jesus our Lord.

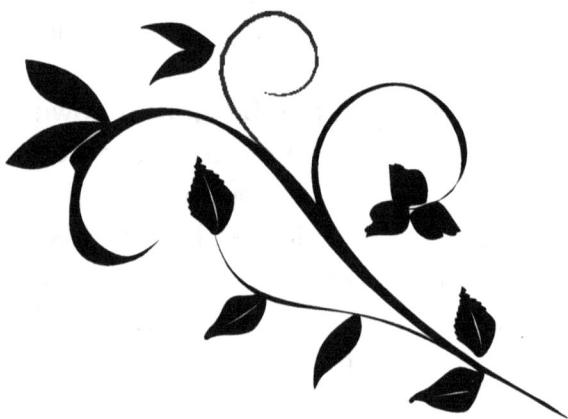

Day 17
Help!

Mom and I were going to visit a friend who'd been placed on hospice. As I got physically ready, I realized I needed to be spiritually ready to offer a word of hope, of encouragement. I know this sweet friend has a firm assurance on where she'll spend eternity. After all, she is one of those who modeled and taught me the faith, one of my Sunday school teachers when I was a teen. Yet, there is sadness about leaving loved ones, about leaving this world.

After my makeup and hair were done, I sat at my desk and turned to the Psalms. Where else? I flipped backward through the book.

150, 149, 148, 147, 146: All beautiful songs of joyful praise we repeat often in our music ministry at the senior village. *Not quite right this time.*

143, *maybe*. Begging God to answer our prayers and deliver us. But, it's talking about reviving. That's not likely for this sister in Christ. Keep a finger here, but look for something more apropos.

139. *Nope.* She's certainly not running from Him—more like stumbling toward Him.

Keep looking, Julie. 136, 135, 134, more praise songs. Not resonating today.

I skipped down a few. 125, 124, 123 too much about wicked scoffers. That's not where we want our thoughts to rest.

122. *So sad*—the reminder she's no longer able to go into the house of the Lord. Definitely not.

Then my eyes lit on 121:

I will lift up my eyes to the mountains;
From where shall my help come?
My help comes from the LORD,
Who made heaven and earth.
He will not allow your foot to slip;
He who keeps you will not slumber.
Behold, He who keeps Israel
Will neither slumber nor sleep.
The LORD is your keeper;
The LORD is your shade on your right hand.
The sun will not smite you by day,
Nor the moon by night.
The LORD will protect you from all evil;
He will keep your soul.
The LORD will guard your going out and your
coming in
From this time forth and forever. (NASB)

That's the one!

Hours later, as I held her hand and read Psalm 121, her lips moved and her tears flowed in joyful recognition. I noticed Mom and our other companions tearing. After all, this passage holds as much value to us—as we face the land of the living. Look to the Lord—expect help from Him. (This reminds me of Jesus' description of the Holy Spirit as *Parakletos*, which can translate as "the Helper.")

He cares. He keeps. He guards and protects our going out, like He has protected our coming in. He's able to keep each of us now and forever. In this world and the next. He's faithful in life, and He's faithful as we pass from death to life (Phil. 1:20-21). That's the help that bolstered my friend—and each of us—in the hospice room.

I pray, my treasured friend, that it bolsters your faith today, as well.

Our Father, please protect our household from all evil; please keep our souls safe in your loving hands. Please guard our going out and our coming in—both on this earth and as my loved one's time of entrance into heaven nears.

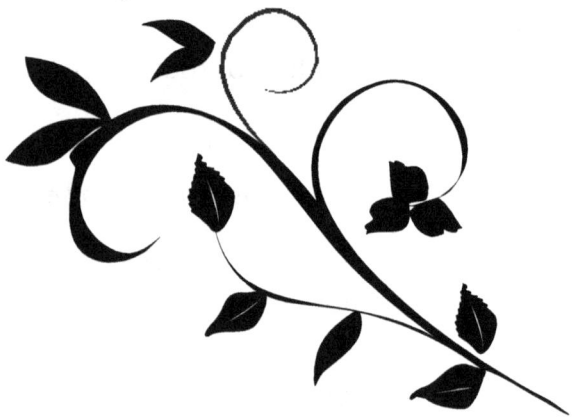

Day 18
Entrusted

Just as we have been approved by God to be entrusted with the gospel, so we speak, not as pleasing men, but God who examines our hearts (1 Thess. 2:4).

When we're not a monolithic club to be courted and manipulated by those seeking not our God but only our vote or our dollars, few outside the faith give much credence to Christians. In fact, truth be told, in greater society it's rather an embarrassment to be a Christian. Add the label evangelical or the term born again, and most of our contemporaries consider us out of step at best and intolerant at worst.

I can't count the times I've been on a plane or train en route to a speaking engagement when my seat mate has struck up a conversation.

"Where are you heading?"

"I'm the speaker at a conference in Dallas (or San Diego or Denver or whatever venue)."

"Oh, I hate public speaking. What do you talk about?"

"I'm also an author, and I'm talking from one of my books."

"People tell me I should write a book. I'll do it some day! Yes I will. By the way, what do you write about?"

Now is the moment I feared would come. *What do I say?* Everything I write centers around Jesus Christ and how He is not only relevant but absolutely essential to life on this planet and safe passage into heaven. As Paul would tell the Thessalonian Christians, that's the message with which we believers in Christ are entrusted.

Notice another key phrase in the opening Scripture verse. "Approved by God." God has vetted us and equipped us to represent the message. We have received His stamp of approval to carry the life-changing message.

When you put it that way ... There really is no way to explain what I do and leave Christ out of the discussion. (Actually, whether we work in secular or religious occupations, there's no way to explain who we are and leave Christ out of the discussion.)

But then there's that rule about avoiding politics and religion in polite society. And there's the real possibility that the word *Christian* will shut down the connection we were building and slam the door on warm conversation for the remainder of the journey.

So, will I mumble with my head down hoping my companion will just drop the issue? Will I appear to be ashamed of the gospel that brings me life and could bring it to my companion, too? Or will I take my chances and speak clearly, "not as pleasing men, but God"?

I know what the apostle Paul's answer would be. In fact, the way the good news of Jesus reached those Thessalonians was a testament to how bold Paul was to speak the gospel without apology. The greater population of Thessalonica was so hostile to the message that the group of believers there had to sneak Paul and his preaching companion Silas out of the city under the cover of night. (For that harrowing story, Acts 17 is a must-read!)

And yet, later Paul was able to write to the church in that city and to say with the utmost truthfulness that he spoke "the message" with "full conviction" (1 Thess. 1:5) among them.

The challenge for us is to speak with full conviction and then to live out the truth in a winsome way among our contemporaries. There, too, Paul and Silas had no reason to be ashamed. In fact, he mentioned to the believers that they knew "what kind of men we proved to be among you." Then he commended them for following his example by becoming imitators of the Lord. He knew this because from them the gospel was going out and touching the surrounding culture (1: 8).

See, it's really not about us. It's about the message sounding across the world. The message that's entrusted to us. The message we're approved by God to carry. He entrusted it to many generations before us. And in each generation, there were those who were unashamed to claim the name of Christ, even to the point of facing death or torture.

The opportunity may come to us in a checkout line or a commuter seat, on a park bench or at a sporting venue, in a hospital elevator, a doctor's waiting room, or at the graveside of a friend. The choice will stand before us—if not today, then certainly tomorrow. In that moment of decision, will I—will you—be unashamed to speak the Truth with full conviction—not as pleasing men, but God?

God, in our quiet moments together, I'm not for a moment ashamed to serve You. To know You. To love You. Help me be gracefully unashamed of Your Name as I go about my business in my sphere of influence today and every day. Keep me alert to opportunities to share your kindness, mercy and love with everyone I meet.

Day 19
Snow Day

*May our Lord Jesus Christ Himself and God our Father …
encourage your hearts and strengthen you (2 Thess.
2:16-17 HCSB).*

We've had a snow day here in our neck of the woods. You'd think that would be rather good, in a way—a time to catch up on lots of stuff we've been too busy chasing around in the outside world to finish. (Come to think of it, I did get a bit of office work in.) But I didn't get nearly as much done as I'd have expected. Although Mom and I did single-handedly (okay, with the help of one shovel between us and one mop handle) attempt to move 500 cubic feet of the white stuff over the side of our deck. We got about two thirds of the way in before quitting in exhaustion. (Don't judge me for letting my senior-citizen mom do such heavy work. She shoved her way into the action with more energy and strength than it would have taken for me to resist her participation!)

In days like these, we find within our energy stores an extra deposit from God—a strengthening for the task that feels supernatural in origin. We certainly felt that as we attacked the snow bank—that is, until we ran up against our physical wall of exhaustion. But, that's the physical and clearly temporary brand of strengthening.

I reread a prayer this morning, from the quill of the apostle Paul, that speaks of a different kind of strengthening—a more permanent one—one that doesn't leave us drained at the end of the experience and collapsing in exhaustion, but instead energizes us for a new kind of future so fabulous that we can't even begin to imagine it. Here it is, found in the closing of his second letter to the Thessalonian Christians.

> May our Lord Jesus Christ Himself and God our Father, who has loved us and given us eternal encouragement and good hope by grace, encourage your hearts and strengthen you in every good work and word (2 Thess. 2:16-17 HCSB).

I pray this Scripture with many of my new students as they enter their writing studies (in part because of the word *word* that makes up a key part of the prayer). But today, I felt very much like the Lord Himself whispered this prayer into my heart—as if the Holy Spirit and the Son of God, who intercede for me always, were praying it for me.

To encourage my heart.

To strengthen me.

To prepare me for the good work He has in store for me.

To open me to the good Word and to the good words (*logos*) He has for me to speak or to write.

Look where this strength and encouragement finds its source: in Jesus Christ and God our Father. And it's based in the love of God for us. It's the source of our hope. And, as I mentioned in the lead-in, it's eternal, perpetual, everlasting, forever, since the world began and after the world ends.

So, I pray this Scripture into your day today—may our Lord, through His love and His Mighty Spirit, show His love for you by giving you an encouragement that will last. So that you may have His hope to sustain you—the hope based in the solid foundation of His promises to you. And may this love and this hope from Him bolster in your heart a firmly planted, growing resolve to keep on with your hard tasks. May it give energy to your tired body—and vibrant life to your tired soul. And may you, now rejuvenated in His strength, do with energy and enthusiasm the work of His calling on your life. May you not only do His will, but speak His words, today and every day.

Oh, and if you happen to be caught in a snow day, be careful moving that white stuff. It looks fluffy and sweet—like cotton candy—but boy-oh-boy can it leave your muscles aching!

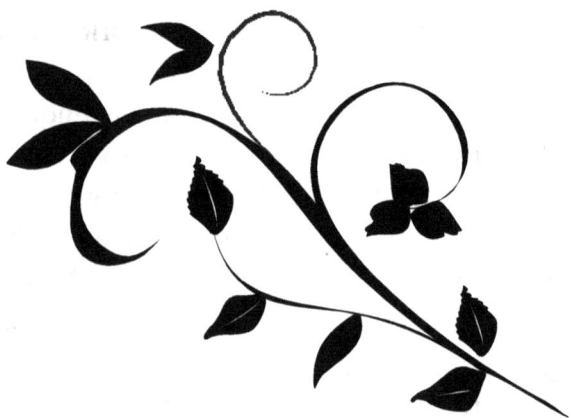

Day 20
Word from My Compassionate Lord

My love will not be removed from you and My covenant of peace will not be shaken (Isa. 54:10).

Leading into each new year, I seek from the Lord a verse of promise, encouragement, even challenge. I reread and review that verse, along with its related passage all year; it provides a growth point for my relationship with Christ. One year, it was John 17—my study of which became my book and Bible study combo package: *Praying Like Jesus.* Other years, the word has been to return to my first love or to simply stand firm when all is falling apart around me. It's a tradition I've kept since college—and one I am continuing this year.

Also, for many years, I've kept Bibles open throughout my home and office (something I learned from reading that Billy Graham does it). Each time I pass the open Bible, I read a verse or a passage. It's getting harder now that I need reading glasses to do this—but I keep a dollar-store pair on each open book, so I have no excuse to pass by without reading. I have one open Bible that I read when I'm brushing my teeth, for example. Another on the printer beside my computer. Another on the makeup table in my bedroom.

It was that third one whose pages got blown around when I was vacuuming one day recently. So, when I looked down at it the following evening, it was open to a passage I hadn't read in a long time ... Isaiah 54.

The passage blew me away, as it related to pains and sadness on my heart. Then I got to verse 10, and realized it was the answer to my prayer for a new year's verse. I share it with you from the HCSB, because it's so vibrant and personal:

> "Though the mountains move and the hills shake, My love will not be removed from you and My covenant of peace will not be shaken," says your compassionate LORD (Isa. 54:10).

So much richness is there. So much promise. I love the adjective He chooses to describe Himself: *compassionate!* A word from my compassionate Lord is one I can't possibly ignore. One that comforts me in a way none other could.

And that promise is so vital in our topsy-turvy days. Though this world may quake and shake and all its foundations crumble, my peace with God through Jesus Christ and my position as beloved in His eyes are secure. Absolutely incredible. Only the Almighty could make that promise and keep it. And He does, and He will.

I challenge you to read this passage for yourself today, perhaps even the whole chapter, and see whether our Lord has a word for you from its riches.

Day 21
Jesus, the Caregiver

John's disciples came for his body and buried it. Then they went and told Jesus what had happened. As soon as Jesus heard the news, he left in a boat to a remote area to be alone (Matt. 14:12-13).

Jesus is sad, grieving, exhausted. He has received word that His forerunner and cousin John the Baptist was brutally beheaded by Herod. In His grief he tries to go away privately to a solitary place, so He boards a boat. And yet the crowd won't let Him go. They are needy. They are demanding. They are persistent. They are quick—for they follow on foot, by land, arriving just as He does by boat. They number into the many thousands (five thousand men, alone, not to mention women and children).

If you or I had been in that situation, I wonder whether we'd have stayed on the boat and put out to another place—even to the middle of the lake—anywhere to get away and mourn quietly.

But not our Lord. Listen for the way eyewitness Matthew records His response:

> When Jesus landed and saw a large crowd, he
> had compassion on them and healed their sick
> (Matt. 14:14; NIV).

He saw their need and set aside His human
weakness to serve them—to meet their needs. All
because of His compassion. Imagine the depth of
love that would allow Him to transcend His grief to
reach out to the people who trudged through the
sands and dust to the solitary place—just to be near
Him. It's a love I confess I don't understand. For
when I'm grieving, I understand the drive to get to
the solitary place—to that point, I'm with my Lord.
But unlike His gracious, loving response—woe to
anyone who gets in the way of my private moments
of sorrow—I demand the right of indulging in a
protracted season of sulky depression.

But not our Lord. He heals. He teaches. He
touches. Because of that overflowing heart of
compassion for His desperate creatures.

The next surprise comes that He keeps on
healing and teaching and touching late into the
evening. Far past His own meal time, and theirs.
The disciples, ever practical, see it, although the
Lord seems to ignore the obvious. Finally, after
trying to signal Him from their perches around the
perimeter, they come up close. They stage-whisper
to Him, "Send the people away. They need food,
and the village shops around here will be closing
soon." Their own stomachs are growling—and they
know just what resources they have—just enough

food for them to have a bite each. A little to share with the Master and the inner circle. But it would be rude to eat in front of the crowd.

Imagine their shock when Jesus commands them, "You, give them something to eat" (v. 16).

What? We have less than enough for ourselves! What are You thinking?

Jesus, the compassionate is also Jesus, the Master. And in His role as Master of the Universe, He takes charge (probably with a disappointed shake of His head at the doltish responses of those who have walked closest to Him all these months). "Bring them to Me," He tells the disciples when they show Him a teensy supply of loaves and fishes. You know the story, Jesus taps into the resources of Heaven to multiply five loaves and two fish to meet and surpass the need—for after everyone is full to capacity, twelve baskets full remain (one for each disciple, ironically).

It's not the supply that makes this story, though. It is the heart of the Master that is so willing to provide for the needs of those who seek Him out. He's still the same, today. Although the food and healing touch may come to us in different forms, all the provision of resources we so desperately need as we care for our loved ones, all of it comes from His willing, compassionate, gracious hand.

Yet (I speak only for myself, now; take from it what you will for your own life) as I receive those resources from Him, I'm tempted to hoard them like the disciples, rather than giving them away like

Christ did. I see only the limits of my abilities—of my resources—and seeing the limits, I'm miserly in releasing them, lest I run out and starve myself. Again, like the disciples. I say, or at least think: Be reasonable, Jesus! You can't expect me to give them what I don't have.

His response echoes down the hall to my office this morning, Bring what you do have to Me. That's when He'll bless it and multiply it and make it more than enough to meet the need around me. But I have to be willing to share. I have to be willing to take on the selfless compassion of the heart of our Heavenly Caregiver—only then will I be the conduit for the Lord's miraculous provision to those around me who desperately need a touch, a word of kindness, and many acts of loving service.

Jesus, the Caregiver of Matthew 14, has much to teach. Today, it was a lesson about selflessness I guess I needed most.

Lord Jesus, thank You for the care You demonstrated to the helpless, hopeless crowd—and to me. Give me a generous heart to share the abundance of provision You've poured into me with all those I touch today.

Day 22
The Waiting Game

But those who wait upon GOD get fresh strength
(Isa. 40:31 THE MESSAGE).

Patience may be a virtue, but it's not one of mine. Yet, today, three of my caregiving friends are developing patience in the waiting room. One sits in her office, but her heart is in another state, awaiting word as her father's life hinges on a surgeon's skill. Others sit stiffly in plastic chairs, sipping burnt coffee from Styrofoam cups, flipping frizzled magazine pages, and stealing glances toward doors labeled: No Admittance. There's nothing anyone can do except pray, which is what I'm doing for each of these friends.

In our waiting room times with Dad, we had mixed experiences. Sometimes we were so relieved to see a smiling surgeon emerge with a smug look of his having cheated eternity on Dad's behalf—at least for the moment. But other times, the tall, debonair surgeon's tears spoke the words even he couldn't bear to form. In all of those moments, the prayers of our loved ones—even those far away—

bolstered and reminded us of God's ultimate goodness regardless of the day's outcome.

I love the way Eugene Peterson paraphrases the familiar Scripture above: *wait upon God … get fresh strength.* It's so vibrant. And so direct. Strength to face whatever. Strength from the hand and nature of a loving God. Just knowing God knows and cares and supports and loves us through these times is immeasurably strengthening. And His strength, like the living water of life He offers at our salvation, is limitless—fresh—sweet.

In case you too have a waiting room in your future, I'd like to share several Bible verses that have become meaningful to me during the many waiting-room hours I've endured as a caregiver. The first two I'll group together:

Isaiah 30:18—The LORD longs to be gracious to you.

Lamentations 3:25—The LORD is good to those who wait for Him, to the person who seeks Him.

I love the truths packed in these descriptions: God is good, He's gracious, He offers fresh strength to those who seek Him. He has a passion to be all that we need. He's good to us, which can make us all the more willing and quick to seek Him.

But best of all is a truth that gives real strength to every believer in the waiting room … is a reminder from 1 Thessalonians 4 that this isn't all there is. We wait, more than anything, for the Son of God, once dead and now alive forever more, to deliver us once and for all and lift us heavenward into His eternal kingdom—alongside all those who have died in Christ. Together we'll be, in that day, more alive than we've ever been, and in perfect health throughout eternity.

So, I pray for you, that the Father of our Lord Jesus would grant you peace and grace in your waiting-room times. I pray for you and your loved ones the assurance that comes from placing your faith in Christ's sacrifice on Calvary. If you have trusted Him, you will find fresh strength in your waiting room—because the Lord of Heaven, your Father, promises to be gracious to you and to be with you always.

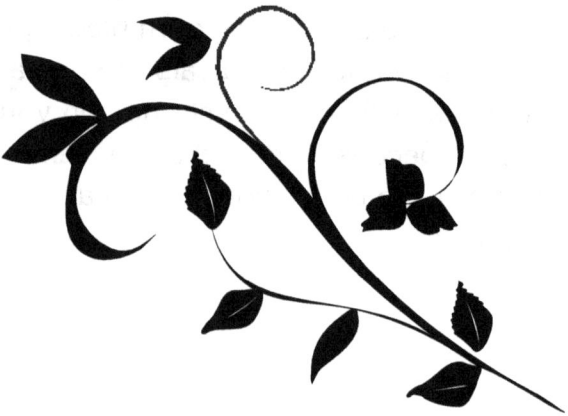

Day 23
Mom, My Best Friend

Then [Jesus] said to the disciple, "Behold, your mother!" From that hour the disciple took her into his own household (John 19:27).

One of the most compassionate and selfless scenes Gospel writers record in the life of Christ occurs in His last moments, as He is gasping for those final breaths. It's a scene I'm thinking about as I write, because in our house gift-giving holidays (like birthdays, Mother's Day, Father's Day and Christmas) aren't single days, but whole-week celebrations. So, Mother's Day ('er week) is on my mind today, although brunch came and went on Sunday.

Here's how John records the scene:

> But standing by the cross of Jesus were His mother, and His mother's sister, Mary the wife of Clopas, and Mary Magdalene. When Jesus then saw His mother, and the disciple whom He loved standing nearby, He said to His mother, "Woman, behold, your son!" Then He said to the disciple, "Behold, your mother!" From that hour the disciple took her into his own household (John 19:25-27).

In honor of my mom, who is my dearest and most understanding cheerleader, supporter and lifelong friend, I have a few observations from the passage that might be both comforting and challenging to those adult children among us who find ourselves cast in the roles of caregiver/advocates for our parents.

The beauty in this scene is three-sided.

But standing by the cross of Jesus is His mother.

The one who didn't always understand Him; didn't always get what He was all about, sometimes even tried to sidetrack Him from the mission His Father sent Him to fulfill—even yet, she stood by Him to the bitter end. The end that pierced her heart, as was prophesied by the sage Simeon on another day in Jerusalem—the day of the infant Christ's dedication at the temple. That's what moms do, at their best.

The second side of the scene's poignant beauty is the Son's action in being absolutely certain that He entrusted the mother He loved into the care of His most beloved and trustworthy disciple—John.

Behold your mother.

In those few words, so much more was said: Take care of this one I love as if she were your very own. Be kind to her. Compassionate. Care for her. See that her needs are met. See that she has safety, protection, food, a place to live, a place where she's needed and wanted and loved. Be to her what

I would be if I were there—companion, friend, confidante. I trust you to do that for her, as if you were doing it for Me.

Don't you love that scene?

Faithful parent. Concerned adult child. Compassionate caregiver.

Eyes meeting, through a veil of tears, in a moment of such intensity that the earth would soon shake in agony and the sky would turn to total darkness.

These are moments we who are caregivers can feel—because in many ways we've been there ourselves. Committing our parent into the care of medical teams, other relatives, staffs at rehab facilities or even nursing homes. Oh, how we can relate to the words of the Son of God—instructing His earthly friend on the long-term care of His mother.

We too have begged—*Care for my parents as if they were your own.*

The final beauty of this scene comes in the simple line,

From that very moment, that disciple took her into his home.

No second-guessing. No waffling about fulfilling the request. No wishy-washy or half-hearted response. An immediate and complete action. Close-up. Affecting John, and Mrs. John, and their entire household. And yet, he did it, out of love for the Master.

Heavenly Father, Help me rededicate myself to doing as John did ... to quickly and openheartedly doing all I can in the care of the loved ones You have entrusted to me–for Jesus' sake.

Day 24
Power and Weakness

"My grace is sufficient for you, for my power is made perfect in weakness" (2 Cor. 12:8).

I want to share with you one of the Scriptures I've been studying lately. I do believe it has direct meaning to each of us in our caregiving roles, as well as to both our ailing loved ones and our personal physical challenges.

It comes from the apostle Paul, and it is an oft-quoted passage—too often, though, quoted at us in our suffering, to chide us rather than encourage us. First, here goes:

> Three times I pleaded with the Lord about this [Paul's thorn in the flesh], that it should leave me. But he said to me, "My grace is sufficient for you, for my power is made perfect in weakness." Therefore I will boast all the more gladly of my weaknesses, so that the power of Christ may rest upon me (2 Cor. 12:8-9, ESV).

First, I observe Paul's emotional pleading to God to remove this debilitating pain from him. Second I observe that God does indeed answer. I guess I'd like to know if God answered Paul when he first prayed, or if He seemed silent until after Paul had pleaded three times. But Scripture doesn't tell us that. It only says Paul got an answer he didn't want, at least initially. God said no to His servant. Here's my paraphrase of what God told Paul: *No, I won't take away this sharp pain that seems to be hindering your ministry. Instead, I'll give you the grace to stand it—and the power to accomplish My purposes in it. Now that you know for sure that you're weak, you'll have the opportunity to see how strong I am.*

I love Paul's response—although it challenges me in my responses. He not only accepts God's answer as sufficient, but he's grateful for the power of Christ that shows itself so clearly in his pain.

Please don't think I'm one of those quoting this Scripture at you. No, I'm sharing it with you, because I've had more than my share of opportunities to live out how true it really is. Even today, I'm feeling painfully aware of my own weakness, yet even so I'm experiencing His inexplicable power to continue my work—in strength that is not my own.

And so, I pray for you today, my friend, that you will experience this same assurance—that even if God answers your prayer by telling you he's not going to change your painful circumstances right now, He will prove Himself gracious to sustain you and powerful to shine through you in them.

I can say this to you only because I know it to be true. And what He did for Paul, what He's doing for me, He's willing to do for you, too.

Day 25
Hefty Price to Pay

One of the most bothersome biblical commands for me has always been the Sabbath rest command.

> Observe the Sabbath day, to keep it holy, as the LORD your God commanded you. Six days you shall labor and do all your work, but the seventh day is a Sabbath to the LORD your God. ... You shall remember that you were a slave in the land of Egypt, and the LORD your God brought you out from there with a mighty hand and an outstretched arm. Therefore the LORD your God commanded you to keep the Sabbath day (Deut. 5:12-15 ESV).

Rest one day in seven. Yeah, right, God, rest? Really? A whole day?

Dad's shots and meds never took a rest. Logging his vital signs didn't take a rest. The need to get his food to him—the right kind at the right time intervals—none of that rested. The ongoing need to make a living so I can, let me see, keep the roof over my head and pay my health insurance every month—that doesn't take a rest. So, how can

I afford to lose an entire day to something as nonessential as rest? When I have the odd moment to actually get some paying work done, I can't be bothered worrying about whether that moment comes around on some other day of the week, or on the day of rest set aside for worshipping the Lord and letting my mind reorder and refresh.

Surely, God, You aren't asking me to rest. Not now! Must be someone else You're talking to about this.

Perhaps that line of thinking sounds familiar.

I was giving that monologue, quite by rote, this morning, as I read the Scripture in my devotions—who says I can't talk and listen at the same time? I'd just completed writing a booklet on the life of one of the last of Judah's kings, Josiah—so my Bible was still open to his story in 2 Chronicles 34. I read past it to the rest of the chronicler's account, where I found a fast-forward report of what happened to Israel's monarchy as Josiah's kids and grandkids, and the people they ruled, ignored God's commands. And I came across this passage that I can't recall ever having noticed quite this way before:

> The LORD, the God of their fathers, sent
> persistently to them by his messengers,
> because he had compassion on his people and
> on his dwelling place. But they kept mocking
> the messengers of God, despising his words and
> scoffing at his prophets, until the wrath of the

LORD rose against his people, until there was
no remedy. Therefore he brought up against
them the king of the Chaldeans. … And they
burned the house of God and broke down the
wall of Jerusalem and burned all its palaces
with fire and destroyed all its precious vessels.
He took into exile in Babylon those who had
escaped from the sword, and they became
servants to him and to his sons until the
establishment of the kingdom of Persia, to fulfill
the word of the LORD by the mouth of
Jeremiah, until the land had enjoyed its
Sabbaths. All the days that it lay desolate it kept
Sabbath, to fulfill seventy years (2 Chron.
36:15-21; ESV).

And here's what jumped out at me:

- Sabbath wasn't a punishment, but a
  privilege. Like all God's commands, it was
  given because of His compassion for His
  people.

- Failure to keep Sabbath had consequences.
  Flouting God's expressed direction, no
  matter which command, meant breaking the
  whole of the law.

- And look at that last verse—the land had to
  enjoy its Sabbaths. God would see to it.
  Witness the utter destruction: the wall, the
  palaces, the precious vessels, even the very

house of God all burned, broken down, uninhabitable.

This fulfilled a promise God made to Moses back in Leviticus, "While you are in your enemies' land; then the land shall rest, and enjoy its Sabbaths. As long as it lies desolate it shall have rest, the rest that it did not have on your Sabbaths when you were dwelling in it" (Lev. 26:34-35; ESV).

Now, the only conclusion we can draw is that for some reason the provision of a one-in-seven (days and years) rest is of vital importance to Him. It's something He built into creation. And it's something that we can't risk ignoring.

It won't surprise you that I'm not ready to shut down my computer and give it a Sabbath year (actually, it would have to be a couple of Sabbath years—I've been in the ministry for thirty-plus years without one; mathematicians, help me out here, that would be how many Sabbath years missed?). But I'm ready to commit to taking a day a week out of the office—away from voicemail, email, blogging, Facebook, Microsoft Office, the whole lot of it.

Maybe it'll be Sunday, traditionally the day of worship for those who celebrate the death and resurrection of Christ—but that's one of the days when Mom and I do our ministry together—so by definition it becomes something other than a day of rest for us. Maybe Saturday, as the Israelites celebrated it back in the chronicler's day. Maybe another day—gasp—when clients are in their offices.

But it seems to me that I'd be well advised (after seeing the price His people paid for ignoring it) to repent, to agree to change my ways, and to do it— as Christ gives me the strength to comply.

Does any of this self-correcting musing ring true for you? If it does, will you take up the challenge to do something about it?

And ... if you don't mind, could I ask you to help hold me accountable to do what I've promised? I'm willing to do the same for you, if you ask.

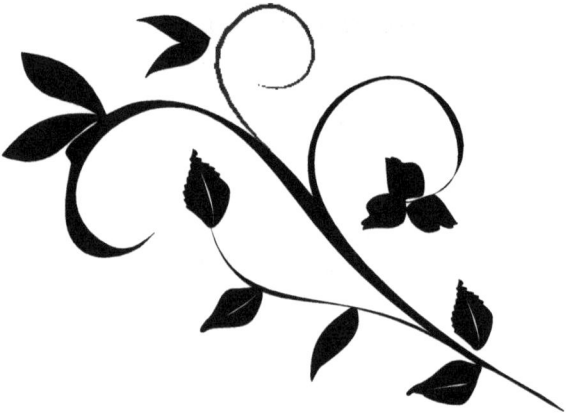

Day 26
Relentless Pursuit of God

As I was reading devotionally in Isaiah 26, a passage ministered to my heart. It seems so relevant to the caregiving journey we are all experiencing. As I read, perhaps you'll see in it what God's Spirit has quickened in my heart today.

> You clear a straight path for the righteous. Yes, Yahweh, we wait for You in the path of Your judgments. Our desire is for Your name and renown. I long for You in the night; yes, my spirit within me diligently seeks You, for when Your judgments are in the land, the inhabitants of the world will learn righteousness (Isa. 26:7-9, HCSB).

The heading for the section in the *Holman Christian Standard Bible* is "God's People Vindicated." And I love that. The injustice and suffering that swirls around us in this world of exhaustion isn't getting the last word. And it isn't as out of control as it feels. God is at work— sometimes, as in the case of His faithful servant Job, His hand clearing a path for our feet is deeply hidden behind the scenes—but He is there, at work and ready to meet the righteous on their path of seeking Him.

I love that the passage gives us a defining picture of the abstract concept of righteousness. It's not sinless perfection—none of us could ever claim that. But it is a passionate desire for God's renown—God's reputation. It is an adoring, zealous seeking of Him—even in desperate times when He seems so tragically far removed from us. A pursuit of Him leads us in the paths of righteousness—the paths that are level and straight. It sounds a lot like Psalm 23: "He guides me in paths of righteousness for His name's sake."

The picture in my mind is of a bruised but persistent hunter: panting, gasping, wheezing through the dark underbrush of a dense forest in the dead of night—even then undeterred because she's hot on the trail of God. Never giving up the pursuit—not when scarred by thorns or thistles; not when chewed up by deep-woods insects; not when tailed by blood-thirsty predators.

I want to be that brand of righteous person, whose path God can ultimately level, as I seek Him that ardently.

As I read and studied further, I went to my *Life Application Bible Notes* on the passage, where I found this comment:

> At times the "path" of the righteous doesn't seem smooth, and it isn't easy to do God's will, but we are never alone when we face tough

times. God is there to help us, to comfort us, and to lead us. God does this by giving us a purpose and giving us provisions as we travel. God provides us with relationships of family, friends, and mentors. God gives us wisdom to make decisions and faith to trust him. Don't despair; stay on God's path.

I suppose I needed that challenge and encouragement this week, as our family suffered the terrible shock of the unexpected death of one of our own elders. As all of you who have suffered a similar loss know, in those hours, we are more obviously desperate for God's face, for His wisdom, for His provision of faith to battle the crouching enemy of despair.

I know this passage encouraged me to keep pursuing God in righteousness, even when I don't understand what He's "up to" in my life, and in the lives of my beloved ones.

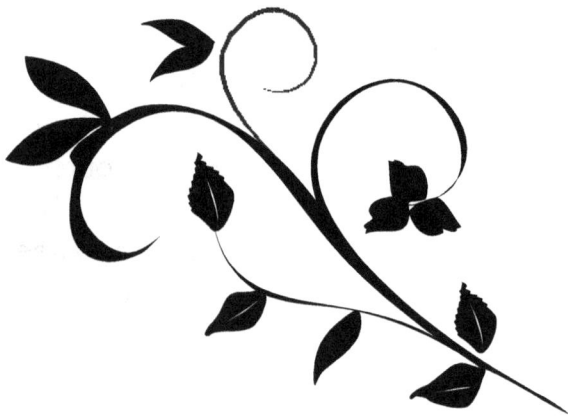

Day 27
The Wind Ceased

Immediately Jesus reached out His hand, caught hold of [Peter], and said to him, "You of little faith, why did you doubt?" When they got into the boat, the wind ceased. Then those in the boat worshiped Him and said, "Truly You are the Son of God!" Matthew 14:22-33 (HCSB)

The setting of this familiar story is that Jesus has stayed behind on land after a busy day of ministry, so He could go alone to talk with His Father in Heaven. He's sent His disciples on ahead by boat. Yes He finally comes walking along on the Sea of Galilee—but only after the disciples have been enduring hours of a storm battering them and threatening to overturn their small craft.

I guess I love this passage so much because I see both what I am (in Peter leaping out in faith, thinking better of it, sinking, and crying out for Christ's help) and what I could be (in Jesus creating a space for His quiet, intimate, personal relationship with His Father in the midst of a chaotic and exhausting season of life).

More often I'm sinking and crying out in desperation than intentionally carving out a time and place for communing with my Father in heaven. Perhaps you are too. Reacting to the crises roiling around you. Leaping out on the water and praying there will be rocks under foot to keep you from drowning—not realizing there was no trick to walking on water—only well-placed, unwavering faith in the Son of God.

I love that Jesus works with the little faith of Peter—and of each of us. Even though He knows how it's going to unfold, He doesn't keep Peter from making the leap. He sustains the miracle so Peter does indeed take a few steps out there on the water (the only human ever recorded to have done so, other than Jesus Himself).

And when Peter's faith peters out (it had to be said), He doesn't say, "Peter, you have no faith, or your faith is of absolutely no use." Just , my friend you have small faith, weak faith, "little" faith—enough to start, which is good (better than the others still cowering in the rocking and rolling boat)—but not enough to finish. It's great, though, that Christ does have the supply of what we lack. He simply reached out and lifted His disciple to safety. And, do note that Peter knew enough to call out for Christ to save him as he sunk into the white caps of the stormy lake.

That, I suppose is the most powerful observation from the scene. Jesus has the power to lift us to safety—not just barely, as if the effort of it will put Him in peril or drain His strength supplies—but plenty of power to lift each of us out of the waves, limitless power, unsappable power, uninterruptible power to carry us to safety in the storm and through the storm. Ultimately, as with the end of this scene, He has the power to overcome and calm the storm—and in so doing to bring honor and glory to Himself. And He is as near to us as to Peter—near enough to hear us when we call; near enough to offer His strong arm to keep us from sinking in defeat.

Another passage I've been reading is from the Gospel of John (chapter 9) where Jesus heals the man born blind—after His disciples want to know whether the man's sins or his parents' caused his blindness. I love that Jesus sluffs off that question entirely and points out that the man's suffering will result in ultimate glory for the Son and His Father in heaven. It's nobody's business what got him there. Only that God has a plan in and through it—one that's good for the man and good for the King's reputation.

That's the way I want to see the storms I'm facing today—through the eyes of faith—even if it's Peter's "little" faith. Even then, it's well-placed faith in the Christ Who not only walks on the water to meet the disciples in the storm, but holds the power to bring them through safely and restore calm to all the forces of nature at work against them.

If you have thoughts on this passage, post a comment: womencareforagingparents.blogspot.com, or drop me an email: conferences@joymediaservices.com. I'd love to know how God is at work in your life through the challenge and encouragement of His Word.

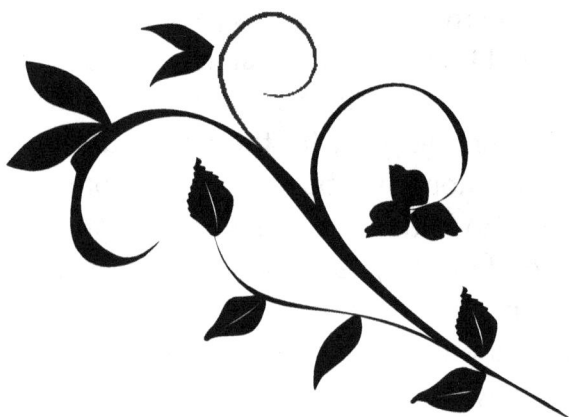

Day 28
Email from God

Therefore let us be diligent to enter that rest, so that no one will fall (Heb. 4:10).

I know that title must sound rather odd—especially coming from me. But I'm pretty sure I received one last week—an email from God, that is.

My work load has been heavy. I've been juggling project deadlines in between shuttling to doctor visits and trying to do my share of household work—including a portion of what used to be Daddy's work before he moved on up to heaven.

It was Thursday around 2 o'clock. I'd been writing all day—about seven hours at that point. That's a pretty intense assignment. And it probably surpassed the wise max for one sitting. But all I knew was I had so much more to get done—it was a rare day without doctors or other interruptions (even the dinner was made already), so I had to capture those hours to move the paying work forward.

The only problem was I was slowing down from fatigue. No, more than that—I was weary to the bone. My head was throbbing. Unconsciously, I brought my hands up to massage my temples. I'm so tired, I moaned.

That's when the email dinged. Now, I'm usually pretty disciplined about letting it ding all it wants and ignoring it until I'm done writing. But for some reason, when my right hand returned to the mouse, I clicked the open mail icon and found the new email. It was a weekly devotional I receive from the Assemblies of God Women's Ministries department—designed especially for Women @ Work. The headline read: *The Rest of Your Life.* And the subhead read: *Coffee Breaks Are Not Optional.*

It might as well have been flashing neon. I read on:

> Learning to work well is great, but working well
> is not sufficient to create a balanced life; we
> must also learn how to stop working. That's
> called rest. ... It was on God's Top Ten List.

You know, I found myself thinking, I may not have too much trouble with some of the commands on that list:

Don't murder—sure, no problem.

Don't steal—okay, what's not mine doesn't belong in my sticky fingers.

Honor your parents—I'm working at that every day and so are you!

Don't take God's name in vain—got it—I love that Name, and will work not to do or say anything that would discredit that Name.

But rest? I'm pretty-much too busy to get that one covered.

Surely, God you didn't mean for me to worry about that one. I'm pretty sure we talked about this one before and decided I was exempt. Right God?

As I read more of the devotional, I was reminded of the command from God that all of us rest—not just on the Sabbath but at other points in our busy days. And I found a bullet-list of warning signs that I'm not up to snuff on that particular command: mental fatigue (check); irritability (check); anxiety (check). Kinda like looking in the mirror.

The emailed article was written by someone I've never met by the name of Ed Gungor. Ed might have written it, but I pretty much consider it an email from God, sent from Ed's keyboard.

So, I did a little homework on rest. I found a great challenge in the book of Hebrews.

> The one who has entered His rest has himself also rested from his works, as God did from His. Therefore let us be diligent to enter that rest, so that no one will fall, through following the same example of disobedience (Heb. 4:9-11).

This passage attributes to God an invitation to His children to enter the gift of His rest. But God I'm doing the Sabbath thing, kinda. Isn't that enough? Then I stopped. No "buts" allowed. I pushed back from the keyboard; shut off the monitor; and went to the family room to rest. Was it convenient?

Nope. Was it in the schedule? Nope. Was it without cost? Nope. Was is necessary? You bet!

I never want to be found on the wrong side of the Word—and when I give account to God one day, I want it to be a joyful moment, not a shameful one.

My prayer is that this challenge will be one we'll take to heart, not just on a Sabbath day, but at regular intervals throughout our week of caring for our aging loved ones.

Day 29
In Oblivion

But as for you, Bethlehem Ephrathah, Too little to be among the clans of Judah, From you One will go forth for Me to be ruler in Israel (Micah 5:2).

I'm fascinated (and sometimes perplexed) by what goes viral on social media. Maybe it's a cute baby (or puppy) doing something darling. Other times it's something troubling done by someone who should know better. Seldom, though, is it an everyday, daily task common to womankind.

Getting up before dawn to trudge out in the snow so we can make the commuter train and get to work on time. Tossing a load of clothes into the washer or running the vacuum when everything in our body screams to be on the couch snoozing after eighteen hours of endless chasing. Preparing a meal for our family when we'd like—just this once—to be served instead of serving. Unless something remarkable happens during these daily comings and goings, not one person takes notice of our sacrifices in these monotonous events.

Laboring in oblivion is where most of us spend our days. Keeping a roof over the heads of our loved ones; being sure they're fed and clothed and well-stocked in necessities. That's where our energy tanks get drained to the dregs.

I see that kind of dailyness when I read Micah's now-famous prophecy about Bethlehem. It's a snapshot of tens of thousands of daily days.

But you Bethlehem ...

An insignificant place, a community of dozens (maybe hundreds) of families keeping flocks fed, baking small cakes of bread in stone ovens, sweeping dust from rocky floors in dark cave-like dwellings, trying to eke a living out of sandy ground.

Too small to be noticed. Too inconsequential to warrant a second glance from outsiders.

But you Bethlehem ...

Even so, for centuries this unassuming place sheltered the remnants of David's kingly line. For, according to Matthew 1's genealogy it was to this tiny place that a young man with that royal birthright and his pregnant bride would be called to return—to his family home. And so would begin a sequence of events that would rock the planet from that generation through ours and beyond.

But you Bethlehem ...

You will shelter the King of kings.

This striking turn of events makes me wonder what eternal significance is taking place in the inconsequential events of our dailyest days? What person are we impacting for the kingdom of God—

simply by a touch on a shoulder, an understanding smile, or a word of comfort? What post on our social media account will encourage a distant friend to keep pressing on for one more day?

But you Bethlehem ...
But you [fill in your name here] ...
Though your day be small and insignificant ... though you toil in oblivion ... though your life seems spent in a million meaningless tasks. Even so, be assured that God sees you and has reserved something remarkable for you. It just may be hiding in a very small package in the Judean countryside of your life.

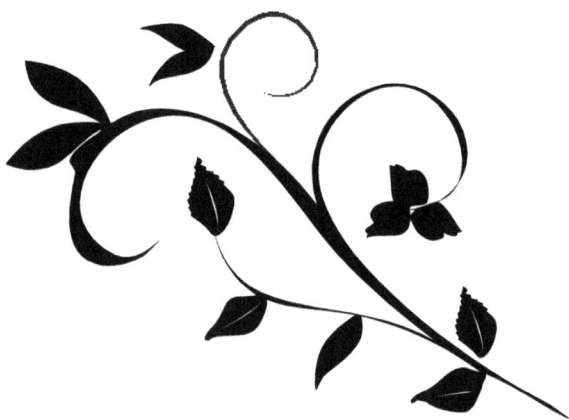

Day 30
A Hope-filled Benediction

I was in the process of preparing for a worship service Mom and I would be leading later in the week. The topic in our series was suffering as Christians. That's why I had my Bible software open to 1 Peter. Peter has a great deal to say about suffering. Suffering for Christ as His examples and His witnesses. Suffering for doing good, rather than as punishment for something wrong we've done. "Give all your worries to God for he cares about you," Peter would write (1 Pet. 5:7). This after acknowledging that Jesus wasn't kidding when He told His disciples, "In this world you will have trouble" (John 16:33).

You know as well as I that we caregivers have become expert in suffering and in trouble of all sorts. It's another of those honorary degrees we definitely don't want but have earned nonetheless.

Suffering calls on us to push aside our bodies' own needs to meet the needs of those more desperately needy than we are. It forces us to sit and watch helplessly as its barbed weed sprouts to full height, hogs all the soil's nutrients, and squeezes out the once-vibrant health of our loved ones.

We see suffering. We experience suffering. We may grow to resent and even despise it. Never, never, never would we consider that it could become something with an eternal purpose. It couldn't possibly be. And yet, that's just what Peter shows us it can become. Here's what Peter said on that note:

> Now for a little while, if necessary, you have been distressed by various trials, so that the proof of your faith, being more precious than gold which is perishable, even though tested by fire, may be found to result in praise and glory and honor at the revelation of Jesus Christ (1 Pet. 1:6-7).

That's nothing short of mind-blowing. Suffering and trouble can become precious like purest gold, because they can showcase Christ's glory and honor? Whoa! What a concept!

As I continued studying the text to share with our congregation, I began looking for the benediction Peter gave on the subject of suffering. Sometimes it helps to see it in black and white on paper, rather than on screen. So, I picked up my leather-bound NLT—which is actually the one I'd given my dad years ago. I remember seeing him pour over it for hours, as he hunched over his desk. I remember delighting in the fact that the Word was coming alive to him in fresh ways because of its contemporary language and turn of phrase. In fact, I should tell you that Daddy highlighted so much of that Bible, that there are few spots on any given page that aren't marked up in some way. Whole sections of it are so well read that they're detached from the spine.

Anyway, the Bible opened immediately to the page I'd been seeking, as Daddy had left a marker (a torn envelope, actually) right in the page where Peter gives the benediction—which, by the way, was absolutely perfect for our congregation that day. And yes, like so many others, this particular passage was highlighted by Daddy's hand. What a heritage he left me.

Here is the benediction I offered for my fellow-worshippers, and it's the benediction—the biblical blessing—I'd like to leave with you beloved caregiver. From the pen of the apostle Peter, recorded in 1 Peter 5:10-11:

In his kindness God called you to share in his eternal glory by means of Christ Jesus. So after you have suffered a little while, he will restore, support, and strengthen you, and he will place you on a firm foundation.
All power to him forever! Amen.

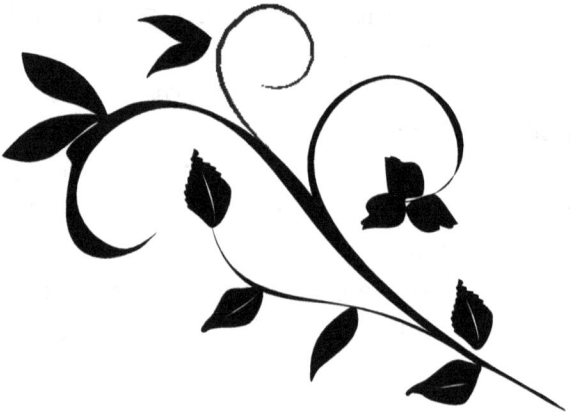

Bonus
Tips for Caregivers

• Even when your loved one is distressed, it's important for you to remain calm, supportive, and controlled.

• Your loved one may become disoriented, frustrated, even angry. But the situation will be less likely to escalate if you remain patient and flexible.

• You can help the patient by maintaining eye contact when she speaks, and by being careful not to criticize, correct, interrupt, or argue.

• Be aware of safety concerns in your loved one's home. For example, remove area rugs and extension cords that could be tripping hazards, disable (or unplug) appliances, and keep household chemicals in an inaccessible place.

• Keep a list of emergency numbers close: doctor, police, fire, ambulance, family members.

- Be on the alert for signs of stress in yourself, and schedule time to take care of yourself. You'll be a better caregiver if you remain healthy and refreshed, in body and in spirit.

- Be willing to accept (and seek) help from others.
- Maintain a journal or a blog to chronicle joys and sorrows. It can be therapeutic to record your thoughts and experiences.

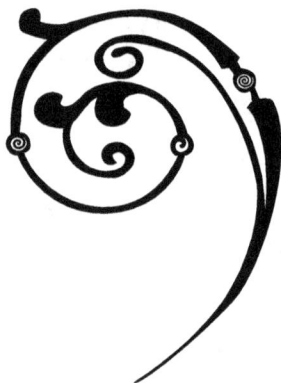

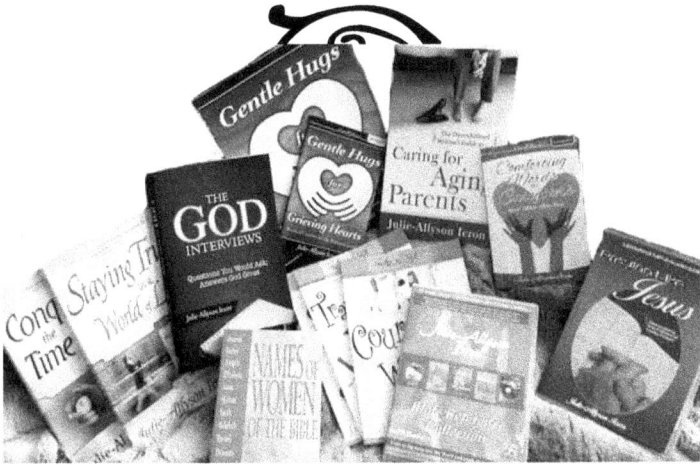

These are just a few of Julie's many titles available on <u>WomenCareforAgingParents.com</u>.

Among the caregiver-specific resources you'll find on our site are:

- Updated caregiver resource list
- Devotional blog links
- Grief devotional and Bible study package
- Free short-reads on self-care
- Dozens of Christian living helps in audio, eBook, and print formats.
- Free short videos from Julie's live-audience and TV presentations, edited to encourage and lift your spirit.

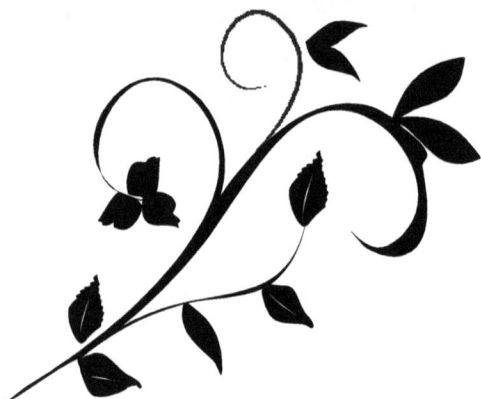

*If we may assist you in knowing more
about Christ and the Christian life,*

*please write
without obligation to:*

joy@joymediaservices.com

*If you benefit personally or spiritually from this study,
please visit* womencareforagingparents.blogspot.com
*and leave a comment for us.
Also visit* womencareforagingparents.com *to
check out our
other products for caregivers and our
additional Bible studies, Christian Living books,
audio productions, e-books, and more.*

*Julie is available to speak for your retreat,
conference, or special event—
whether your group is large or small.*

To check date availability, write to:
conferences@joymediaservices.com